Lecture Notes in Biomathematics

Managing Editor: S. Levin

67

Philip H. Todd

Intrinsic Geometry of Biological Surface Growth

Springer-Verlag

Berlin Heidelberg New York Tokyo

Author

Philip H. Todd
Department of Anatomy, Dundee University
Dundee DD1 4HN, Scotland

Mathematics Subject Classification (1980): 92-XX

ISBN 3-540-16482-0 Springer-Verlag Berlin Heidelberg New York Tokyo
ISBN 0-387-16482-0 Springer-Verlag New York Heidelberg Berlin Tokyo

Printing and binding: Beltz Offsetdruck, Hemsbach/Bergstr.
2146/3140-543210

T A B L E   O F   C O N T E N T S

CHAPTER 1

INTRODUCTION

1.1 General Introduction

The work which comprises this essay formed part of a multidisciplinary project investigating the folding of the developing cerebral
cortex in the ferret. The project as a whole combined a study, at
the histological level, of the cytoarchitectural development concomitant with folding and a mathematical study of folding viewed from
the perspective of differential geometry. We here concentrate on
the differential geometry of brain folding. Histological results
which have some significance to the geometry of the cortex are referred to, but are not discussed in any depth.

As with any truly multidisciplinary work, this essay has objectives
which lie in each of its constituent disciplines. From a neuroanatomical point of view, the work explores the use of the surface geometry of the developing cortex as a parameter for the underlying
growth process. Geometrical parameters of particular interest and
theoretical importance are surface curvatures. Our experimental
portion reports the measurement of the surface curvature of the
ferret brain during the early stages of folding. The use of surface curvatures and other parameters of differential geometry in
the formulation of theoretical models of cortical folding is discussed.

Generalized from its neuroanatomical context, we are to analyze the
relationship between growth and intrinsic geometry or 'shape' of a
biological surface. Our object from the standpoint of mathematical biology is to define a methodology for analyzing the change in
intrinsic geometry during biological growth. In parallel to this
essentially biometric function, a general methodology for modelling
surface growth processes will be suggested.

The major challenge and principal difficulty of communication, whether verbal or written, is to present in some logical but strictly sequential order the essentially non-sequential products of the intellect. In a study whose motivations are as diverse as this, any imposed sequential order must be to some extent arbitrary. The following is the order used.

The remainder of the introduction, as an overture, picks out the major themes of the ensuing chapters and provides a setting in the respective disciplines of neuroanatomy, computer geometry and mathematical biology. Chapter 2 presents a number of case studies where differential geometry is used as a parameter of biological surface growth. These studies serve both to introduce the vocabulary of classical differential geometry in a biological context and to lay the theoretical groundwork for the neuroanatomical observations of chapter 4 and the theoretical mathematical biology of chapter 3. Chapter 3 presents a general intrinsic surface growth model. In conjunction with this model, a metric for intrinsic surface shape difference is derived. Chapter 4 presents the results of surface curvature measurement during the early stages of folding in the ferret cerebral cortex. These curvature measurements are related to the underlying cytotechtonic growth processes.

While multidisciplinary in its scope, the style of this essay is intended to be such that it is of interest to the non-specialist biologist or mathematician. In some sections this means parallel arguments are given: a non-technical account of the mathematical problems tackled and models formulated, and a rigorous mathematical exposition of these models. An exception to this rule is the appendix on numerical curvature estimation: here the problems encountered are internal to the numerical analysis and as such of little interest to the nonmathematician.

The structure of the monograph is problem oriented inasmuch as it follows a sequence of ideas focused on the measurement of brain curvatures. This sequence represents an introduction to biological differential geometry; the formulation of a general mathematical model for biological surface growth; an exposition of the data extraction and analysis techniques for curvature estimation; results and discussion of an experiment to measure the curvature of the ferret brain.

Background material to the diverse segments of the thesis comes
from the literature of several distinct subjects. It is therefore
appropriate to structure the remainder of this introduction by
disciples. In effect, two different introductions will merge to
impinge on the body of the text: one from the direction of mathematical biology, and a second from neuroanatomy. The confluence of
these different valleys of ideas, we hope, should leave a rich al-
luvium for intellectual growth.

1.2. Introduction from Mathematical Biology

Mathematics impinges on Biology in two distinct areas: the formulation of models of biological systems in mathematical terms - this
is the realm of 'mathematical biology' or 'biomathematics'; the application of high technology to biological measurement and the
interpretation of data thus obtained - this activity may be
labelled 'biometrics'.

Some mathematical techniques have traditionally lent themselves preferentially to one or other of these activities. Differential equations have been used widely in biological modelling: examples are
numerous and include Volterra-Lotka predator-prey models, reaction
diffusion models for morphogenesis, Hodgkin-Huxley nerve axon
model. For a general view of differential equations in biology see
Jones & Sleeman (1983). Harmonic analysis, on the other hand, has
been applied mostly in data gathering and interpretation. Examples
include the decomposition of time dependent data streams, such as
ECG's and EKG's into harmonic components for subsequent analysis
and diagnosis, the reconstruction of a tomograph section from a
subset of its projections (Crowther et al. 1970), harmonic analysis
in an attempt to classify shape, either performed mathematically
(e.g., Younker & Ehrlich 1977) or optically (Scheiben 1979). For a
critique of the latter application of harmonic analysis see
Bookstein et al. (1982).

The subject of this essay is the use of differential geometry in
biology. The applications discussed intersect both the spheres of
biomathematical modelling and the extraction of biometrical parameters. In particular, we are interested in the relationship

between growth and the geometry of a biological form. We will be seeking both geometrical models for certain growth processes and suitable geometric parameters for measuring such processes. First we discuss some general properties of geometrical shape parameters, then look at some approaches to biological growth modelling.

Shape Parameters

In chapter 3 a metric will be proposed for the difference in intrinsic geometry between Riemann surfaces. In order that we are able to assess this particular parameter as a quantification of intrinsic shape difference, it is appropriate to examine the role of parameters in a more general context. In particular, we shall look at the difficulties involved in quantifying geometrical concepts, such as shape.

Much of experimental science involves attempts to measure the effect of a 'treatment' on some property of an experimental system. The first requirement is that a measurable parameter of the system be quantified. The selection of this parameter is governed by the particular property of the system which is under study. The shape of a biological object, as perceived by a trained observer can be an important diagnostic and experimental variable. The shape and texture of a stained cell reveals much about its structure and function to the trained cytologist. The shape of a leaf may enable the botanist to classify a plant. In comparison with the complex discrimination of shape achieved by the human visual system and its subsequent analysis by the trained observer, the parameters commonly used to quantify shape seem crude indeed. An example of these parameters is the long diameter/short diameter ratio, which is a measure of eccentricity; a similar parameter is (long diameter)^2/area; (perimeter)^2/area is a commonly used measured of circularity.

Despite the necessary crudity of any quantification of shape in comparison with human perception, there are two reasons for persisting in attempting to quantify shape. In order to implement automated diagnostic systems, for example automatic screening of cervical smears for cancer cells, it is desirable to emulate the expert's

perception of cell size and shape by computer. The machine's decision process, in contrast to the human's must be overtly quantitative: quantitative shape parameters are therefore required. At a
different level, if a statistical analysis is to be made of a shape
property, then some quantification (perhaps only a ranking) of
shape is required by the statistics. In an analogous way, the mech-
anistic procedures by the statistics and image analysis both require quantitative input, although they usually generate a qualitative output.

The shape of an object may be defined to be the collection of its
geometrical properties which are invariant under similarity transformations. Hence a parameter which purports to quantify shape
must be invariant to change in scale, position and orientation.
For this reason shape parameters are dimensionless. A single shape
parameter, such as those mentioned above is only able to describe
one particular aspect of the overall geometry of an object. It is
therefore essential to select a parameter which is as sensitive as
possible to the particular shape property which is of interest and
is as insensitive as possible to the other factors which influence
overall shape. A parameter may be called a shape parameter if it
is invariant to change of scale and orientation. The equivalence
classes of parameter are fundamentally connected with the nature of
the property which it quantifies.

Growth Modelling

Two strategies are available for the modelling and measuring of biological growth. The first strategy is to analyse a biological form
as a network of discrete points, usually landmarks identified
either directly anatomically or by geometric construction from anatomical landmarks. Growth is then seen as a distortion of the network, is characterized by a finite set of extensions of the edges
of the network, and is susceptible to multivariate analysis. For a
review of work of this type see Humphries et al. (1981). This approach is useful in some practical biometric problems such as
cephalometrics (Walker & Kowalski 1981), numerical taxonomy
(Strauss & Bookstein 1982). For the purposes of modelling the

biological growth process, however, it is perhaps more appropriate to take an analytic view of growth.

An analytic description of growth treats and finite change of form as the integral of infinitesimal differential growths throughout the biological form. Such a treatment puts biological growth into the province of continuum mechanics. The language of continuum mechanics, suitably adapted to emphasize differential material growth rather than externally applied force as the dominant driving force, is now applicable. For a review of work on analytic growth models, along with a clear exposition of the laws of continuum mechanics as applied to such models, see Skalak et al. (1982). Examples of continuum growth models are Richards and Kavanagh's (1943, 1945) early work on tobacco leaf, further analysis of the same leaf by Erickson & Sax (1956), more plant growth models by Erickson (1976) Silk & Erickson (1978, 1979). Models of tip growth include work on fungal tips (Green 1969, DaRiva Ricci & Kendrick 1972), and on root tips (Hejnowicz & Nakielski 1979). A more general model for growth within plant organs is found in Hejnowicz (1982).

The methodology outlined by Skalak et al. (1982) traces the position during growth of material points in the plant or animal under study. If we let a_i be the coordinates at the time t_0 of specific (in theory identifiable) points of the biological form.

If $R = aa_i$, then R is the region of space occupied by the form at time t_0.

If $x_i(t) = x(a_i, t)$ are the coordinates of these points at the time t, then $X(a_i) = x_i(T)$ for some fixed T represents the growth transformation of the initial form R to a new form $R_T = X(R)$. A key parameter of this transformation is the 'growth extension tensor' e_{ij} defined by

$$\frac{(dS)^2 - (dS_0)^2}{(dS)^2} = e_{ij} da_i da_j$$

where dS_0 and dS are the initial and final lengths of a line

element da. The growth extension tensor thus defined is analogous
to the material strain tensor of conventional continuum mechanics.

Growth, then, may be seen as a form of material strain. The mathematical structure of biomathematical growth problems is, in a
sense, the dual structure of the typical stress-strain problem of
solid mechanics. In the latter problem, the strain tensor typic-
ally represents the response of the material to some externally applied stress. In the static problem, an equilibrium configuration
of the solid is sought which balances externally applied stress
with restorative forces which are the product of the material under
strain. The dynamic problem represents the response of the solid
to changes in the external stress. In a typical biological growth
problem, on the other hand, applied stress may play no significant
part in the process. The dynamic behaviour of the system is a response to change in the material strain due to growth; the right
hand side of the stress-strain equation has been altered, and a new
equilibrium configuration is required to balance the (presumed constant) external stress.

Mathematically there is little difference between adapting material
configuration as a response to strain change and adapting it as a
response to externally applied stress. Biological growth models
do, however, appear rather strange to the practitioner of orthodox
solid mechanics. Conservation of mass is a central assumption to
most physical and engineering modelling. A body which is free of
unbalanced external forces will behave in an inertial way. Growing
biological systems however, contravene this basic tenet. Left to
itself, a biological system may add mass and grow. Of course, the
laws of physics are conserved, the added mass comes from whatever
nutrient the animal or plant is imbibing. The most appropriate
model may, however, represent the animal or plant itself as a
closed system; within that system mass is not conserved.

A further dissimilarity between the continuum mechanics of biological growth and physical solid mechanics lies in the complexity of
the applied influences. A classical problem of solid mechanics is
modelling the strain on a loaded member. Although the distribution
of strain through the member may be complicated and intricately dependent on the geometry of the member, the applied stress may be
due simply to a unidirectional gravitational force, with perhaps

compression or extension of the member. The external influence
applied to a growing biological form, on the other hand, may be a
spatially ordered regime of differential growth controlled by some
unknown but sophisticated morphogen. The complexity of the regime
of growth may be essential; it thus may be that the system does not
admit a simply physical analogue model.

The analytical description of growth given by Skalak et al. (1982)
is continuous in space and time. For some studies, where frequent
data sampling is not possible, for example in phylogenetic growth
studies, finite growth mappings are studied. In such cases, for
example D'Arcy Thomson's (1942) famous method of transformed co-
ordinates, or Bookstein's (1978) biorthogonal grids, comparison of
related forms constitutes a growth analysis. A mapping or 'coordinate transformation' between initial and final form is interpolated
from landmarks on the form. The study of growth is then a study of
mapping between two regions of Euclidean space representing two
stages in the growth process. D'Arcy Thomson's original coordinate
systems are arbitrary: one form has a cartesian grid imposed, the
other form has a curvilinear coordinate system. Bookstein removes
this degree of arbitrariness by stipulating a 'biorthogonality'
condition: each superimposed grid must be orthogonal. This, he
shows, defines a unique pair of grids on the two forms.

The problem of determining an appropriate mathematical map between
two biological forms, in the absence of landmarks, is tackled in a
different context by Schwartz (1977, 1980). His mapping is not a
growth mapping; it is the retino-tectal map of the goldfish visual
system. The shape of the retina and the tectum impose geometrical
boundary conditions on the map; without interior landmarks, however, further postulates are required. For this system, Schwartz
claims that appropriate further assumptions are that the mapping is
conformal, and that the average magnification factor is minimal.
With these assumptions, the required map is the solution of a
classical Dirichlet problem and thus is wholly determined by the
boundary conditions, which are prescribed by the geometry of the
retina and tectum. This strategy is appealing: the biological
nature of the forms to be mapped guides the selection of an appropriate mapping. The selection criteria take the form of a re-
striction on the class of maps to be considered (conformal maps),
and a minimisation principle. Minimisation principles may

frequently be connected with the geometry of region boundaries via some form of Green's Theorem. Such a model has the clear advantage of mathematical tractability. It's vulnerability to criticism is from a biological standpoint - on the applicability of its axioms. The main function of a mathematical model - to force attention on some critical well-defined properties of the modelled system - is thus fulfilled.

In many biological models, some boundary between regions of different structure is of critical importance. It is appropriate in such cases to use the language of surface geometry to model the material interface. In Greenspan's (1976) tumor growth model, the interface is that between the tumor and its surrounding nutrient; the geometry of this surface determines in the model the local rate of uptake of nutrient. In a model of Skalak et al. (1982), bone grows by the secretion of material at its surface. Some biological forms, either because of their thinness or because of their laminar structure, may be treated as mathematical surfaces. An example is a surface tension model of the alveolus (Dimitrov et al. 1982). The cerebral cortex, we shall argue, may be regarded as a growing surface. It is appropriate, then, that the subject of this essay is surface growth modelling.

The normal force due to surface tension is proportional to the average curvature of the surface. Hence an important parameter of the dynamic interaction between a physical surface and its surrounding medium is the surface average curvature. The mechanical importance of this parameter is reflected in several models such as D'Arcy Thomson's (1942) cell surface tension models, also in his minimal surface analogies for the shape of radiolaria. Models where average curvature assumes a significance independent of surface tension include Greenspan's (1976) aforementioned tumor growth model; Sinai et al. (1982) postulate that moisture content of semi-arid soil is proportional to average curvature of the field, Louie & Samorjai (1982) model the alignment of DNA and RNA strands in terms of paths on minimal surfaces.

From a mathematical point of view, Gaussian curvature is a more important parameter than average curvature. Gaussian curvature is invariant under isometry: surfaces whose geometry changes from the viewpoint of the embedding 3-dimensional space, but whose internal geometry does not change, retain the same Gaussian curvature. This property is exploited in the discussion of Van Essen & Maunsell's (1980) paper on cortical mapping; this paper will be referred to further in our neuroanatomical introduction.

To summarise the biomathematical aims of this work: we shall investigate surface growth models of biological systems. In particular we shall attempt to formulate a general model for biological surface growth and to derive parameters for such growth which are sensitive to the interplay between extrinsic and intrinsic geometry.

1.3 Neuroanatomical Introduction

The cerebral cortex comprises an external layer of the brain; it has a laminar structure. It is widely recognised that the basic functional units of the cortex are columnar arrays of neurons through the depth of the cortex (Rakic 1981). Again, the fundamental developmental subdivision of the cortex is the developmental column (Todd & Smart 1981). Among species of the same family, smaller species tend to have smooth brains, whereas larger species have folded brains. For example, while most smaller rodents have smooth brains, the Capybara has a folded brain (Campos & Welker 1976); while many prosimians have simple folded brains, the smaller prosimian Tarsius Spectrum, for example, has a smooth brain (Radinsky 1968). The usual measure of the cortical capacity of an animal is the surface area rather than the volume of its brain (Jerison 1963, Sacher 1970). It is the allometric relationship between the requirement for the cortical capacity to grow as a surface and the volumetric growth of the brain itself which creates the need for folding in larger species. These observations all point to the appropriateness of treating the cortex as a mathematical surface.

This essay will investigate surface geometric aspects of the cortical folding process. The animal used for this study is the ferret. The ferret is an attractive animal for several reasons: it is a small inexpensive laboratory animal, the cerebral cortex has a simple folding pattern which is, nevertheless representative of a large class of carnivore brains, finally, folding takes place postnatally, thus a developmental series covering this period may be easily acquired. The ferret is used as a model for the effect of neurotoxins on the brain development (Haddad et al. 1975); it is thus important to have a good description of normal growth in this animal. Of course, we hope that the observations made in the ferret are more generally applicable outside the species.

We here briefly report some histological observations, properly part of the companion histological study, which are pertinent to our geometrical arguments. We then look at two competing views of the interrelationship between growth, function and cortical folding; we define a geometrical experiment to distinguish between these two models.

The ferret is born at approximately 42 days post conception. Neuron production is concentrated between 22 and 38 days p.c. By birth, the cortical plate is essentially complete in terms of cell number, it is of uniform thickness and histology. Folding takes place between 2 and 20 days post partem, and coincides with growth of the cortical plate through cell maturation and the addition of intercellular processes. No significant increase in the number of neurons in the plate takes place at this time. Before folding, the histological structure of the cortical plate is uniform, there is no histological indication for the site of presumptive folds. The appearance of a non-homogenous cytoarchitecture, however, coincides with the onset of folding. The cortex at the bottom of sulci is very much thinner than elsewhere in the cortex, the columnar streams of cells are less apparent, and the classical cortical layers apparently merge (Smart 1984).

A point of some interest is the causitive relationship between these two contemporal phenomena: the establishment of regional cytoarchitectural differences and the folding of the cortex. Is the differential thickening of the cortex the manifestation of some basic regional cell-structural, and eventually functional different-iation, and do the mechanical or other properties of this regional differentiation cause folding to follow its spatial patterns? On the other hand, does the folding process itself cause a realignment of otherwise uniform tissue and are the resulting apparent differ-ences in cytoarchitecture merely differences in spatial assembly of cells, in no way indicative of intrinsic cytoarchitectural or functional differences.

The above impinges on the question of whether the folds have functional significance. Even a speculative answer to this question is not straightforward. The rhinal fissure is a special fold, present even in smooth brains, and clearly marks the boundary between paleocortex and neocortex. Many other sulci are traditionally used to delineate boundaries between functional regions of the brain, for example the central sulcus and lunate sulcus in primates reliably delimit the motor area and visual area respectively (Connolly 1950). Physiological studies on a variety of species (e.g., Walker & Campos 1963, several species of the family Procyonidae; Campos & Walker 1976, on the Capybara) apparently identify some folds as 'limiting' sulci between different functional regions of the cortex, others as 'axial' or central to functional regions.

A functional significance for folding is implicit in phylogenetic interpretations of skull casts of monkeys (Falk 1978), of hominids (Radinsky 1974), of canids (Radinsky 1973 b), and of carnivores (Radinsky 1971). In these studies casts of animal or fossil skulls yield folding patterns. The folding patterns together with an assumption that folds retain a constant position with respect to functional regions across a phylogenetic timescale are used to construct a history of differential brain specialisation during evolution. The analysis depends crucially on the constancy of the position of folds with respect to functional regions. The ambiguity of the results in this field, the absence in general of histological techniques and the ambiguity of physiological results make it unclear whether the majority of folds have functional significance.

Two cortical folding models have assumptions which broadly correspond to the two views of the functional significance of folds. Le Gros Clark (1945) postulates folding as a response to the mechanical stresses caused by spatial differences in the physical structure of the cortex. The folds may either be between areas with different properties (`limiting sulci') or at the centre of such an area ('axial sulci'). The reason why such regions possess different mechanical properties is the actual cytoarchitecture is developing differently, and thus, we assume, the presumptive function of the regions is different. Richman et al. (1975) postulate a

mechanical model for folding, driven by differential elasticity
between layers of the cortex, but assuming transverse uniformity.
Their model thus tends to follow the uniform growth picture of
folding.

Van Essen & Maunsell (1980) also view folding as growth of a uniform cortex with an isometric deformation (bending but no shearing)
generating the folds. While constructing flat maps of cat and
macaque cortex, they discover that 'only modest distortion' is required. This is interpreted as loosely indicating that the folding
process has not introduced too much differential stretching of the
cortex. They identify two distinct elements in the folding process:
the first they call 'pure folding'; by which they mean the crump-
ling or folding of a surface which undergoes none but uniform
growth. To avoid confusion with the whole process of convolution
formation, which we call folding, in this work we will call this
special case 'isometric deformation'. The second component of the
folding process, Van Essen & Maunsell call 'intrinsic curvature';
this is folding accompanied by differential growth.

> 'It is of interest to know the relative importance of
> folding versus intrinsic curvature in accounting for the
> convolutions of the cerebral cortex. There is obviously
> some intrinsic curvature associated with the wrapping
> around of the cortex to form an almost completely enclosed
> surface, but the question is whether the formation of
> convolutions results in a major increase in intrinsic
> curvature....'
>
> Van Essen & Maunsell (1980).

Evidence of major increase in 'intrinsic curvature' is evidence for
differential growth, hence for differential form of neurons and
hence differential function correlated with the folding process.
If folding is all isometric, then we have nothing to dislodge the
theory of a uniform cortex with functional regions and folds in-
dependently superimposed.

Van Essen & Maunsell identify Gaussian curvature and average curvature as important parameters of the folding process. Gaussian
curvature is invariant under isometry. Under a uniform growth plus
isometric deformation regime, Gaussian curvature will decrease as

the inverse square of the linear growth. If differential growth is present Gaussian curvature will behave in a different manner. Average curvature is seen as a measure of 'pure folding'.

The neurobiological objective of this essay is to test the hypothesis of Van Essen & Maunsell by measuring surface curvature of the ferret brain during the early stages of folding. Further we postulate and test a theoretical link between the overall surface geometry of the brain and the pattern of folding superimposed on it. Having measured surface curvatures, we expect to be able to assess how much differential growth is present during folding, and to say something about the spatial distribution of the growth.

CHAPTER 2

SOME GEOMETRICAL MODELS IN BIOLOGY

2.1 Introduction

In this chapter, we address the dual tasks of introducing the basic
concepts of differential geometry on which subsequent arguments
will rest, and of exploring at a basic level the major thematic
areas of our subsequent development. A sequence of five case
studies will be presented, in each of which surface geometry plays
a crucial role as a morphological parameter. The elementary concepts of differential geometry will be introduced as needed in
these case studies. The studies are ordered by the complexity of
the mathematics required.

The shape and growth of many biological forms can be treated as surface phenomena. We consider surfaces which manifest themselves as
submanifolds of 3-dimensional Euclidean space; that is the normal
space of everyday life. The shape of such surfaces may be viewed
in two different ways; either from the perspective of the three
dimensional space in which they are embedded, or from the limited
'intrinsic' perspective of the surface itself.

As an example let us compare the geometry of a flat sheet of paper
with that of the same sheet of paper rolled into a half-cylinder
(fig. 2.1.1). Viewed from the embedding 3-D space, the shapes of
flat sheet and half-cylinder are obviously different. The distance
between points A and B in fig. 2.1.1, measured on the sheet is L.
When measured in the embedding 3-dimensional space, however, the
distance is $2L/\pi$. If we constrain ourselves to remain in the sheet
itself, however, although the path is now curved, the distance between A and B is still L. In fact the intrinsic surface geometry
of the sheet has not been altered by bending it. Geometry on a

cylinder, when we restrict ourselves to remaining on its surface, is therefore the same as geometry on a flat sheet.

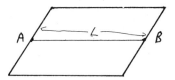

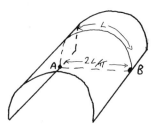

Fig. 2.1.1. A flat sheet retains its intrinsic geometry when rolled into a cylindrical shape.

A familiar example of curved surface geometry is that of the sphere. The distance between Edinburgh and Dunedin from a naviga- tional point of view is not the straight-line distance through the earth's core, rather it is the length of the shortest path (or 'geo- desic') which joins the two cities while remaining on the surface of the earth. The fact that the earth cannot be mapped faithfully on a 2-dimensional chart, has given rise to a variety of different projections, each of which represents some geographical features accurately, while distorting others. This necessary distortion is due to differences in intrinsic geometry between the sphere and the plane.

Shape is the fundamental parameter of morphology. As real biologi- cal surfaces are always observed in a 3-dimensional context, it might seem that the intrinsic view of shape is too restrictive. However, we shall attempt to show that in certain biological sys- tems, it is the intrinsic, or 2-dimensional geometry of a surface which can yield important clues to the phylogenetic or ontogenetic processes which dictate its resultant form. As we are interested in the interplay between growth and shape, we shall be looking largely at biological forms in pairs rather than individually. Our main interest, then will lie in analysing shape change in order to elucidate the various processes underlying the change.

Corresponding to the two different perspectives of surface geometry referred to above, we identify two types of shape change: firstly change in the three dimensional shape of a surface without any change in its intrinsic geometry and secondly change in the intrinsic geometry of a system. It is the way which geometric change can reflect change in the biological structure of a surface and its interaction with the surrounding medium which is of primary interest. A change in the intrinsic geometry of a surface must be accompanied by some change in the biological or physical properties of the surface itself: at least some areas must stretch or shrink. (This is similar to the need to distort when making a flat map of the earth). This change may or may not be accompanied by changes in the surrounding medium. On the other hand, purely extrinsic shape change, unaccompanied by change in intrinsic geometry (such as rolling up a sheet of paper) may be achieved purely by changes in the extrinsic factors affecting the surface, and with no change in the structure of the surface itself.

A case of particular interest is that where changes in the surface itself can be assumed to be substantially or entirely responsible for the shape change. For example, the shape of a leaf is determined by the cellular structure of the leaf itself, and not by any great extent by the pressures exerted on it by the surrounding atmosphere. Less obviously, in many biological systems, although patently affected by the nature of the surrounding medium, the surface may be the dominant biological feature. We shall assert in the sequel that the cerebral cortex is such a system: that it is events within the cortex which control its geometry, rather than external influences such as pressure of the skull or of subcortical white matter.

In such cases, change in intrinsic geometry can be a useful parameter for growth. A qualitative example of this approach is the following. Observation of the change in surface geometry when a bud grows out from a plant stem may suggest that there is local growth in the plant at the place where the bud appears. This conclusion is not reached from observation of the cell kinetics per se, but from a prior knowledge that such a change in surface geometry, from a cylinder to a cylinder with a hemispheric bud, is associated with local growth in the region of the bud.

As a further example: the observation that in primates, the frontal lobes of the brain are more prominent than in, say, carnivores suggests differential phylogenetic growth of the cortical areas at the front of the brain. This deduction is not based on direct measurement of the size difference between functional areas, but from a qualitative assessment of the relation between the change in shape of the brain and the underlying growth causing that change.

The 'deductions' of the previous two paragraphs are ad hoc and only qualitative. It is part of the objective of this and the next chapter to work towards a systematic quantitative approach to the analysis of the relationship between differential surface growth and shape change. We will largely, although not exclusively, be concerned with situations where the surrounding medium plays no obvious part in determining the shape of the object under study.

It is hoped that this thesis should be intelligible to both the general mathematician and the interested biologist. An attempt will therefore be made to keep parallel strands of argument going: on the one hand, a rigourous mathematical treatment, on the other a verbal description of the analysis, which is in general intuitively appealing and raises some questions of biological interest. For the benefit of the non-specialist, we shall quietly introduce the tools of of differential geometry while discussing a number of disparate biological case-studies. In the next chapter we shall attempt to formulate a general approach to the analysis of biological shape change.

2.2 Hemispherical Tip Growth

Tip growth, whether root tip (Erickson 1966, Erickson & Sax 1956), hyphal tip growth in fungi (da Riva Ricci & Kendrick 1972), or general plant apical cell growth (Green 1965, 1969, 1976), is a biological problem with a high geometrical content. It is well known that in these cases growth is localised at the tip; the simple geometry of the system has enabled a number of analysts to derive the distribution of growth from the geometry under a variety of assumptions as to the nature of the growth.

The geometry of tip growth is appealing, and lends itself to mathematical modelling. The most common model is of a cylinder of non-growing 'set' material capped by a hemispherical tip or apex of growing material. This geometry remains constant as new material is added at the tip, and the cylindrical stalk is, as a result, elongated. Different simplifying assumptions as to the type of growth then lead to different quantitative models of the differential growth in the tip.

We shall, after introducing the mathematics necessary to an appreciation of this subject, discuss these different models. We shall present our own re-solution of one of these models, less from an intention to contribute to the study of tip growth than to explore a methodology which is capable of generalisation.

Summary of the mathematics

The geometric subject of this essay is a 2-dimensional surface embedded in Euclidean 3-dimensional space; that is a surface which is capable of real life manifestation. (A Kline bottle is a familiar example of a 2-dimensional surface which requires a 4-dimensional space to live in.)

A mathematical surface has no depth. A real-life surface is therefore usually the boundary between two 3-dimensional spaces: for example the surface of the earth is the boundary between the solid earth and its atmosphere. Where a physical object has negligible depth, for example a sheet of thin paper, we tend to regard it as a surface, although to be strict we should specify whether our surface is the top or bottom of the sheet or perhaps some internal boundary.

The most convenient way to treat a surface mathematically is in terms of two parameters which define a coordinate system on the surface. The coordinate system thus formed is called 'curvilinear' as

the coordinate grid lines are in general not straight lines. A
familiar example of a curvilinear coordinate system is the lines of
latitude and longitude on the earth's surface.

Having defined a surface parametrically, a crucial question is:
how does parametric distance on the surface relate to Euclidean
distance in the embedding 3-dimensional space. On the earth's surface, the question is: if someone travels for 1 degree of latitude
or longitude, how far has he gone. This example demonstrates the
complexity of the question. If someone at the equator travels 1
degree of longitude, he will have gone 1/360th of the earth's circumference. Again if he travels through 1 degree of latitude, he
will have covered 1/360th of the earth's circumference. If however
someone at a higher latitude makes the same two journeys, he will
find that a journey of 1 degree latitude north or south still takes
him through 1/360th of the earth's circumference, a journey of 1 degree of longitude, east or west, will only take him through 1/360th
of the circumference of that particular line of latitude. Close to
the pole this distance could be very short indeed.

The 'first fundamental form' of a surface performs the task of
relating parametric distance on a surface to real distance. It is
in fact in general a tensor quantity; this means that its effect
can be different in different directions (as seen in the above
example). The first fundamental form 'contracts' with any unit
vector to give a scalar distance in the direction of the unit
vector.

Our interest in growth forces us to look not at single surfaces but
at growth mappings between surfaces. Growth may then be quantified
by the ratio of distance on the new surface to distance on the old
surface. That is the ratio between the first fundamental form contracted in a particular direction on the new surface and the first
fundamental form contracted in the corresponding direction on the
old surface.

A case of particular interest is where the ratio between first
fundamental forms is the same in all directions. In this case
growth is said to be 'isotropic' and is quantified by a scalar
growth factor - the ratio between first fundamental forms. In
biological terms the meaning of isotropy is clear. If a small

circle were drawn on the growth surface, the radius of the circle might increase, but it would remain a circle. Anisotrophic growth, on the other hand, implies the existence of a directional preference; the small circle would grow more in one direction than the other and become distorted in growth to an ellipse.

The analysis of this section will focus on a model of tip growth. The geometry of the model is as follows: a hemispherical growing tip surmounts a cylindrical non-growing 'stalk'; throughout growth the geometry remains the same, new material is added at the tip and the resulting growth causes the stalk to be elongated.

This geometry alone is not sufficient to specify the growth; two further assumptions are made. The growth is assumed to be both radially symmetric and isotropic. With these assumptions, it is possible to equate growth parallel to and perpendicular to the axis of the stalk (isotropy implies equal growth in both directions). Growth perpendicular to the axis is predetermined by the geometry and, because of isotropy, dictates the growth parallel to the axis. We can thus achieve a quantitative description of the growth undergone by the tip.

Tip Growth Models

Green (1965) follows Erickson & Sax (1956) in analysing tip growth in terms of so called 'Relative Elemental Growth Rates'. These are measures of instantaneous growth over the tissue and are defined as follows:

Let $h(t_1)$ be the length of a particular linear element and the surface at time t_1, and $h(t_2)$ its length at time t_2. Then the ratio of first fundamental forms of initial and final surfaces, or 'growth factor', in the direction of the linear element is:

$$\lambda = h(t_2)/h(t_1);$$

this growth has occurred in time $(t_2 - t_1)$.

To obtain some 'average growth factor', it is convenient to take logs, so

$$\log(\lambda) = \log(h(t_2)) - \log(h(t_1))$$

an average rate of growth would be:

$$\frac{\log(h(t_2)) - \log(h(t_1))}{(t_2 - t_1)}$$

and an instantaneous rate

$$\frac{d\log h}{dt} = \frac{1}{h}\frac{dh}{dt}$$

This is termed the relative elemental growth rate.

If g(t) and h(t) are the lengths of perpendicular linear elements on the surface, then the area growth rate is identified as:

$$\frac{1}{gh}\frac{dh}{dt}\frac{dg}{dt}$$

Green studies three types of model. His first model forces area growth rate to be constant over the surface; shape change is achieved by varying degrees of anisotrophy. This model he labels 'isokinetic'. The antithesis is the isotropic model, where shape change is driven by differential growth. He synthesises these extremal models to produce realistic analyses of biological structures.

Da Riva Ricci & Kendrick solve the isotropic model numerically.

In this chapter we shall present a re-solution of the isotrophic model in a form which we shall later extend into a general methodology for analysing biological shape change.

The Mathematics of Axisymmetric Growth

There are several different schemes of notation for differential
geometry. The appropriateness of each scheme depends on the degree
of generality and the depth to which the subject is to be explored.
The level used here is roughly that of Struik (1950). Following
him the notation used will where possible by the Gibbs form of
vector analysis. Tensor notation will usually be avoided; it is
felt that the advantages of more concise mathematics are outweighed
in these applications by the further barrier imposed by the use of
tensor notation between the non-specialist and the meaning of the
mathematics.

We shall define our surfaces parametrically as the following locus
of points in Euclidean 3-space Cartesian coordinates (x, y, z):

$$(x(u, v), y(u, v), z(u, v)) \text{ for } u_1 < u < u_1 \text{ and } v_2 < v < v_2$$

or in vector notation as $\underline{x}(u, v)$.

The distance element ds = $d\underline{x}$. $d\underline{x}$ may be expressed as follows:

$$ds^2 = (\underline{x}_u du + \underline{x}_v dv) . (\underline{x}_u du + \underline{x}_v dv) \tag{2.2.1}$$

where

$$\underline{x}_u = \frac{\partial x}{\partial u} \text{ and } \underline{x}_v = \frac{\partial x}{\partial v}$$

or

$$ds^2 = Edu^2 + 2Fdudv + Gdv^2 \qquad (2.2.2)$$

where

$$E = \underline{x}_u \cdot \underline{x}_u \quad F = \underline{x}_u \cdot \underline{x}_v \quad G = \underline{x}_v \cdot \underline{x}_v$$

Equation (2.2.2) is called the first fundamental form of the surface.

Our interest is in surface growth. We restrict ourselves here to considering growth in discrete time intervals, mainly because the biological system we shall be most interested in, the cerebral cortex, only admits viewing at discrete time intervals. Such growth may be characterised by a mapping from one surface (the initial surface). This 'growth mapping' takes each point on the initial surface onto its destination point on the final surface.

Let S be the surface $x(u, v)$ and S_1 be the surface $x_1(u, v)$ where

$$x_1(u, v) = \varphi(x(u, v))$$

The mapping ϕ is isotropic if $ds_1 = \lambda ds$

For our axisymmetric growth model, we require the growth map ϕ to be both isotropic and axisymmetric.

Let S be a simply connected surface, symmetric about the z-axis, with boundary ∂s. We look at the curve in the x-z plane which generates S when rotated about the z-axis. Parametrise this curve:

$$(f(s), z(s)) \text{ for } 0 \leq s \leq s_1$$

Now if we parametrise surface S by s and θ, then

$$S = (f(s)\cos\theta, \; f(s)\sin\theta, \; z(s)) \quad 0 \leq s \leq s_1; \; 0 \leq \theta \leq 2\pi$$

Let T be another simply connected surface with boundary ∂T, symmetric about the z-axis and with generating curve

$$(g(t), \; w(t)) \text{ for } 0 \leq t \leq t_1$$

then

$$T = (g(t)\cos\theta, \; g(t)\sin\theta, \; w(t)) \quad 0 \leq t \leq t_1: \; 0 \leq 0 \leq 2\pi$$

An axisymmetric mapping : $S \to T$ induces a function $t(s)$ such that

$$\varphi(\underline{x}(s, \; \theta)) = \underline{x}(t(s), \; \theta)$$

If in addition, φ is isotropic then there is a scalar 'growth factor' $\lambda(s)$ defined at each point s and

$$2\pi f(s)\lambda(s) = 2\pi g(t(s)) \tag{2.2.3}$$

This is the growth factor acting in the direction transverse to the axis of symmetry.

Also

$$\int_0^s \left[\left(\frac{df}{d\sigma}\right)^2 + \left(\frac{dz}{d\sigma}\right)^2 \right] \lambda(\sigma) d\sigma = \int_0^t \left[\left(\frac{dg}{dr}\right)^2 + \left(\frac{dw}{dr}\right)^2 \right] dr \qquad (2.2.4)$$

This is the growth factor acting along the axis of symmetry hence

$$\frac{dt}{ds} = \frac{\left(\frac{df}{ds}\right)^2 + \left(\frac{dz}{ds}\right)^2}{\left(\frac{dg}{dt}\right)^2 + \left(\frac{dw}{dt}\right)^2} \frac{g}{f} \qquad (2.2.5)$$

The differential equation (2.2.5), along with boundary condition

$$t(s_1) = t_1 \qquad (2.2.6)$$

yields a unique t and along with this unique conformal map φ. The growth factor $\lambda(s)$ may be obtained from equation (2.2.4)

$$\lambda(s) = g(t(s))/f(s) \qquad (2.2.7)$$

Tip Growth

We specialise now to the tip growth problem. The geometrical model is of a truncated sphere mapping onto a hemisphere (figure 2.2.1).

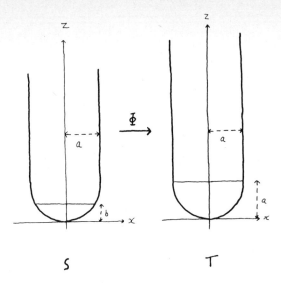

Figure 2.2.1. Tip Growth Model

Let surface S be the truncated sphere

$$(2as - s^2\cos\theta, \quad 2as - s^2\sin\theta, \quad s) \quad 0 \le s \le b$$

S has a radius a and is truncated at z = b. Let T be the hemisphere:

$$(2at - t^2\cos\theta, \quad 2at - t^2\sin\theta, \quad t) \quad 0 \le t \le a$$

then from (2.2.4)

$$\frac{dt}{ds} = \frac{2at - t^2}{2as - s^2} \qquad\qquad (2.2.8)$$

with boundary condition : t(b) = a

whence

$$t(s) = \frac{2as}{2aA^2 + s(1 - A^2)} \qquad (2.2.9)$$

and, from (2.2.7) :

$$\lambda(s) = \frac{2aA}{2aA^2 + s(1 - A^2)}$$

$$(2.2.10)$$

where logA is the constant of integration.   Substituting the boundary condition t(b) = a yields :

$$A^2 = b/(2a - b) \qquad (2.2.11)$$

Equation (2.2.10) gives the local growth undergone by point s on surface S during the transition to surface T.   Growth rates may be read off the formula.   For example if markers are placed a small distance h apart at a point on the tip distance b from the apex, their separation when they have been displaced onto the cylindrical stalk (i.e., when b maps onto a) is :

$$\lambda(b)h = \frac{ha}{b(2a - b)}$$

$$(2.2.12)$$

These are the displacements determined numerically by da Riva Ricci & Kendrick (1972).

Summary

The importance of tip growth as an illustration is that from the geometry of the system, along with some simplifying assumptions about the nature of the growth process, it was possible to derive an expression for the differential growth of the surface. This is exactly the theme which will be generalised in chapter 3.

2.3 The Mouse Cerebral Vesicle

Our second case study applies the mathematical development of section 3.2 to an entirely different biological system. A simple geometric model of the development of the mammalian cerebral vesicle will be analysed. Differential growth factors, derived from the model, will suggest a link between the spatial patterns of differentiation in the tissue and the geometry of the growing system.

In the mouse, at 9 days post conception, the neural tube may be regarded as a simple cylinder of epithelial tissue. The cerebral vesicles develop as a pair of outgrowths from the lateral walls of the cylinder. At this stage (10 - 11 days post conception) the tissue comprising the walls of the vesicles consist of pseudostratified epithelial neuronprecursor cells.

Subsequent events in the development of this area of tissue involve the release of neurons from the precursor epithelium and the aggregation of these cells in the cortical plate, a transitory structure at the pial surface of the vesicle. Both these events have a high degree of spatial organisation. Our model will focus on the early stages, when the geometry of the vesicle is being formed, and while the tissue is simple in its cytoarchitecture. The geometric model for the growth of the vesicle presents some interesting correlates with the spatial organisation of developmental 'events' through the organ. These correlates will be explored after the model is presented.

The geometry of the early stages of vesicle formation is modelled in the following way. The area of tissue on the neural tube of the 9 day embryo which will grow to form the vesicle is modelled as a flat disc. The vesicle itself is regarded as a hollow sphere truncated where it joins the tube (fig. 2.3.1). The growth process is assumed to be axisymmetric about an axis perpendicular to the centre of the flat disc. This forces the centre of the disc to map onto the 'pole' of the vesicle (A in fig. 2.3.1). Isotropy is also assumed.

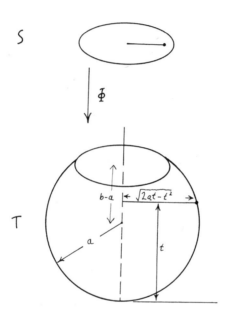

Fig. 2.3.1.   The disc → truncated sphere model.

Mathematical Model of Vesicle Development

Let S be the disc of unit radius:

$$(s.\cos\theta, \; s.\sin\theta, \; 0) \quad 0 \le s \le 1.$$

Let T be the sphere, radius a, truncated at z = b :

$$(\ 2at - t^2\cos\Theta, \quad 2at - t^2\sin\Theta, \ t) \ 0 \leq t \leq b$$

Assuming an axisymmetric, isotropic map from S to T taking the boundary of S onto the boundary of T, we have from (2.2.5)

$$dt/ds = (2at - t^2)/as \tag{2.3.1}$$

whence

$$t = 2aA^2s^2/(1 + A^2s^2) \tag{2.3.2}$$

again logA is the constant of integration.

Substituting t(1) = b yields :

$$A = \sqrt{\frac{b}{2a - b}} \tag{2.3.3}$$

Now from (2.2.7) :

$$\lambda(s) = 2aA/(1 + A^2s^2) \tag{2.3.4}$$

Or, in the coordinate system of the sphere,

$$\lambda(t) = A(2a - t) \tag{2.3.5}$$

As at the 'pole' of the vesicle (t = O) λ = 2aA. At the 'equator' of the vesicle (t = a), λ = aA. Our simple model would therefore suggest that material at the pole of the vesicle has grown twice as much since the flat disc stage as that at the equator.

If we assume that growth is solely due to cell division, this suggests that cells at the pole of the vesicle have undergone 1 more cell cycle than those at the equator during vesicle formation. The synthesis of geometric model and cell production model has some interesting interpretations in the light of Smart's (1983) work on the early development of the brain. These interpretations will be discussed below.

As in the root tip example, we have here built a model for the differential growth of the tissue based solely on an idealisation of its geometry. This type of model, which uses surface geometry as a parameter of growth, is the major theme of this essay.

Morphogenesis and Differentiation in the Mouse Cerebral Vesicle

In the mouse nervous system, onset of neuron production in the cerebral vesicles is preceded by a period of ventricular surface growth which expands the area of ventricular epithelium. During this early stage of development, mitotic figures within the neuroepithelium are arranged so that their planes of cleavage are perpendicular to the ventricular surface, (Smart, 1973), with the result that cell divisions produce increments to the surface area of the ventricle. These geometrical constraints force the ventricular cells to grow and, when neuron production commences, to differentiate as a surface epithelium.

Neuron birth, as determined autoradiographically, is first observed in the cerebral vesicles at about 11 days post conception, signalling a change in the behaviour of the ventricular layer from being a proliferative compartment producing an expanded ventricular surface, to a differentiating compartment producing a proportion of non-mitotic cells which migrate towards the outer surface of the cerebral vesicle. There is circumstantial evidence to indicate that these non-mitotic cells migrate radially following the observed fibre projections from the ventricular surface, and accumulate in radial assemblies (Levitt & Rakic 1980, Rakic 1981). The released cells later form the cortical plate, a transient compartment of immature neurons which, in most mammals, reveals a pronounced radial structure. The radial constraints on migration imply that the ventricular epithelium projects preneurons to the outer surface of the vesicle, and if this interpretation is correct, the appearance of preneurons provides a record of changes in the behaviour of the underlying ventricular epithelium (Smart & McSherry, 1982).

It is evident, both from autoradiographic labelling studies, and from light microscopical studies of the embryonic cerebral vesicles, that neuron production is not uniformly distributed over the vesicles; neurons are first observed opposite the interventricular foramen in a small zone which spreads rapidly over the surface of the vesicle (Smart 1973, 1983). This localised origin and rapid spread of the area of neurons raises a number of interesting questions about the behaviour of the ventricular epithelium, and in particular about the factors controlling the localised switchover from proliferation to neuron production.

Our geometric model of vesicle growth requires a specific regional distribution of growth throughout the tissue. As mentioned above, the release of neurons from the cells lining the vesicle appears to follow a precise spatial pattern. An economic model for the control of this pattern of differentiation links it to the differential growth required to generate the geometry of the organ.

We thus propose the following simple model. The decision for a precursor cell in the wall of the cerebral vesicle to form a neuron is controlled by some mechanism that involves counting elapsed cell cycles since the beginning of vesicle growth. Meanwhile, the geometry of the physical growth of the vesicle is determined by a scheme of differential growth rates imposed on the wall of the neural tube. This difference of growth rates staggers the onset of differentiation over the vesicle, and generates the observed spatial-temporal pattern of neuronogenesis.

In more detail, we make the simple assumption of exponential cell growth. Cycle times are assumed to vary spatially through the process of vesicle formation. This variation in cycle times results in differential growth rates which in turn generate shape change. A spatial variation in the number of elapsed cell cycles over the tissue also results.

Under these simple assumptions, the number of cells in a particular lineage is 2^T, where T is the number of cycles elapsed. Assuming an isotropic structure to the tissue, the amount of areal growth should be proportional to the number of cells input,

$$\text{i.e.,} \quad \lambda 2 = k 2 2^T \qquad (2.3.6)$$

The linear growth is therefore

$$\lambda = k 2^{T/2} \qquad (2.3.7)$$

hence

$$T = 2 \log_2 (\lambda/k) \qquad (2.3.8)$$

It T_e is the number of cycles elapsed at the equator, and λ_e the growth at the equator and if logs are taken to base 2 for the rest of this section then:

$$T - T_e = 2 \log (\lambda/k) - 2 \log (\lambda_e/k) \qquad (2.3.9)$$

$$= 2 \log (\lambda/\lambda_e) \qquad (2.3.10)$$

$$= 2 \log ((2a - t)/a) \qquad (2.3.11)$$

If we then specify that after T_d cycles, the precursor cells begin to produce neurons, we can predict that neuron production will start at the pole of the vesicle t = 0 and spread radially through the tissue. As the pole is 2 cycles ahead of the equator, the time for this spread should be approximately 2 cell cycles.

Figure (2.3.2a) shows the theoretical spread of precursor-neuron differentiation, figure 2.3.2b (from Smart 1983) shows the observed spread of the cortical plate. (The cortical plate is an aggregation of neurons, precursor to the cerebral cortex; the formation of cortical plate is a reliable indicator of the onset of differentiation in a particular region of the vesicle). The time taken for the plate to spread from pole to equator is of the order of 20 - 30 hours (Smart 1983). The cycle time for mouse neural epithelium at 13 - 14 days post conception is about 12 -15 hours (Korr 1980). This agrees closely with the predictions of the model.

Our model was simplistic both geometrically and biologically but, and this is the entire point of such models, it admitted quantitative analysis. The possibility of a link between morphology and the geometry of differentiation is provocative. More important from the point of view of this thesis is the central role of change in surface geometry of the vesicle. The geometry alone suggests that tissue at the pole of the vesicle has expanded most; this suggests that more cell division has taken place there. The observation that differentiation starts on the lateral wall of the vesicle opposite the foramen suggests a link between the onset of differentiation and the amount of cell division undergone by a particular region of tissue.

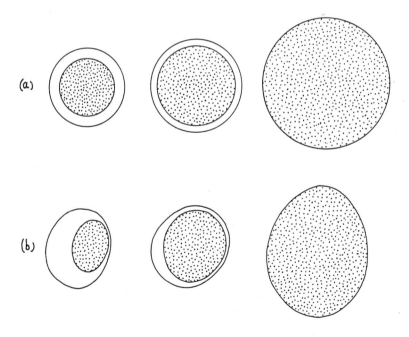

Fig. 2.3.2 (a) predicted spread of differentiation at 1/, 1 and 2 cell cycles after its start; (b) observed spread of the cortical plate on the mouse cerebral hemisphere between 13 and 14 days post conception.

As in the root tip example, the geometry of a mathematical model for a particular biological surface growth determined 'growth factors' for that surface. This regime of differential growth was then used in a model linking the geometry of the developing tissue with the geometry of the spatial spread of differentiation through that tissue.

2.4 The Shape of Birds' Eggs

In this section we introduce the important concept of surface curvature. We introduce this concept in the context of a simple model of the formation of birds' eggs originally proposed by D'Arcy Thomson (1943). This particular biological system is chosen as an example for two specific reasons. First, the surface geometry of the mature egg is used as a parameter of the physical system which generated that shape. As such the example is in the mainstream of the intellectual development of this thesis. Secondly, eggs have a non-trivial surface geometry, which is nevertheless very close to axisymmetric. Their shape is therefore interesting but relatively easy to treat mathematically.

The model of egg formation proposed by D'Arcy Thomson is of an elastic membrane filled with an incompressible fluid. The shape of the egg is caused by the interplay between the external pressure exerted on the membrane by the walls of the oviducts, the surface tension of the membrane itself and the internal hydrostatic pressure of the fluid.

The effect of the hydrostatic pressure of the enclosed fluid is a uniform outward force normal to the surface of the enclosing membrane. The membrane is assumed to be under a uniform surface tension. Under these circumstances, the inward force exerted by the membrane depends on the curvature of the surface. The external pressure exerted by the oviduct on the pre-formed egg must supply the difference between these two forces. This is determined by the curvature of the egg. As the force exerted by the oviduct is also produced by elastic tension, this force is determined both by differential tension and by the curvature of the oviduct, which is assumed to mould itself round the egg and thus adopt the egg's curvature at corresponding points.

In our mathematical development, we shall concern ourself primarily with the definition of the curvature of a surface. In fact there is more that one useful curvature parameter defined on a surface. In this section the important parameter is Average Curvature. Other measures of surface curvature will be discussed at length in following sections.

The radius of curvature at a point on a curve in 2 dimensions is a familiar concept on which we shall ground our discussion. It is the radius of the circle which 'just fits' the curve at that point. Curvature is defined to be the inverse of radius of curvature. A circle of radius, r, for example, has curvature $1/r$; a straight line has curvature 0.

We now consider a surface in three dimensions. At any point A on the surface, the intersection between a plane P normal to the surface at that point and the surface itself, is a curve passing through A. The curvature of this line at A is a curvature associated with the surface at A in the direction of the plane P. A different plane P will yield a different curvature at A.

Of particular interest are those planes P which yield maximum and minimum values for the curvatures. The maximum and minimum curvatures k_{max} and k_{min} and the directions on the surface associated with them will play an important part in the description of the geometry of surface growth.

The Average Curvature at a point on a surface is defined to be the average of maximum and minimum curvatures: $H = (k_{max} + k_{min})/2$. At every point on a cylinder of radius r, the maximum curvature is $1/r$ and is in a direction perpendicular to the axis of the cylinder. The minimum curvature is in a direction parallel to the axis and is 0. The average curvature is therefore $1/2r$. A sphere of radius r has curvature $1/r$ in all directions, its average curvature at any point is therefore $1/r$.

Mathematics

If $\lambda = \dfrac{dv}{du}$ the curvature on the surface in direction $\dfrac{dv}{du}$ is

$$k = \frac{e + 2f\lambda + g\lambda^2}{E + 2F\lambda + G\lambda^2}$$

(2.4.1)

(Struik 1950) Maximum and minimum values of k occur when $\dfrac{dk}{d\lambda} = 0$. It can be shown that in these cases k satisfies the following equation:

$$(EG - F^2)k^2 - (gE - 2fF + Ge)k + (eg - f^2) = 0$$

(2.4.2)

where E, G and F are as defined above (in 2.2.2) and

$$e = \frac{(\underline{x}_{uu},\ \underline{x}_u,\ \underline{x}_v)}{EG - F^2} \qquad\qquad f = \frac{(\underline{x}_{uv},\ \underline{x}_u,\ \underline{x}_v)}{EG - F^2}$$

(2.4.3)

$$g = \frac{(\underline{x}_{vv},\ \underline{x}_u,\ \underline{x}_v)}{EG - F^2}$$

where $(\underline{x}_{uu},\ \underline{x}_u,\ \underline{x}_v)$ is the vector triple product $\underline{x}_{uu} \cdot (\underline{x}_u \ \char94 \ \underline{x}_v)$

If kmax and kmin are the roots of (2.4.2) then the average curvature H is

$$H = \frac{1}{2}(k_{max} + k_{min}) = \frac{gE - 2fF + Ge}{EG - F^2}$$

(2.4.4)

Gaussian curvature, kmax . kmin $= \dfrac{eg - f^2}{EG - F^2}$

(2.4.5)

A Model of Egg Formation

The importance of curvature in this example is due to the fact that the normal force exerted by an elastic surface under tension is proportional to the average curvature of the surface.

D'Arcy Thomson's model for egg formation balances the hydrostatic pressure of the fluid inside the egg against the surface tension force exerted by the membrane surrounding the fluid and the external pressure exerted on the membrane by the walls of the ovary. The hydrostatic pressure of the internal fluid is assumed to be uniform; thus the shape of the egg, and in particular its average curvature yields the differential force exerted on it by the walls of the ovary.

D'Arcy Thomson's equations are as follows. If $p(s)$ is the normal pressure exerted by the oviduct at point s on the egg shell membrane, then $p(s) = P - TH(s)$, where P is the hydrostatic pressure of the fluid, T is the tension in the shell membrane, and $H(s)$ is the average curvature of the egg-shell at s. If p is caused by an isotropic tension T_w in the wall of the oviduct, then

$$T_w H = P - TH \qquad\qquad\qquad (2.4.6)$$

$$T_w = P/H - T \qquad\qquad\qquad (2.4.7)$$

Assuming a static situation a graph of $1/H$ is a graph of the relative tension in the walls of the oviduct along the axis of symmetry.

To apply this model, it is necessary to have a geometrical representation of the egg's surface. We do this in two ways.

Our first approach follows Preston (1953) and Smart (1969) in approximating the egg's outline by a low order deformation of a sphere. Our second approach involves approximating the egg's outline using cubic splines. This more ugly technique admits generalisation to axisymmetric shapes which are less regular than eggs.

Equations for the egg via Coordinate Transformations

Eggs are axisymmetric. We can therefore characterise their geometry by a function describing the outline of a plane section of
the egg taken through the axis of symmetry. We take as a 'base
structure' the circle

$$x^2 + y^2 = 1 \qquad\qquad (2.4.8)$$

We allow coordinate transformations of the form $X = x/a$: $Y = y/af(X)$. (fig. 2.4.1)

Our transformed circle has equation

$$X^2 + Y^2 = 1 \text{ or } x^2 + y^2/f(x)^2 = a^2 \text{ or } y = af(X)\sqrt{1 - \frac{x^2}{a^2}} \qquad (2.4.9)$$

Some transformations : $- f(X) = k = b/a$: yields the ellipse

$$\frac{x^2}{a^2} + \frac{y^2}{b^2} = 1$$

(i) $f(X) = k + cX$ gives the standard 'ovoid' described in Preston (1953).

The equation for the ovoid is :

$$x^2 + \frac{y^2}{(k + c\frac{X}{a})^2} = a^2$$

(ii) $f(X) = k + cX + dX^2$:- describes some eggs which are 'aberrant' when fit to linear transformations.

(iii) $f(X) = k + cX + dX^2 + eX^3$:- the cubic term is brought in to adequately describe eggs such as that of the guillemot.

(iv) $f(X)$ - higher order :- the success of low order transforma-
tions in describing egg geometry precludes the need for higher order approximates to $f(X)$.

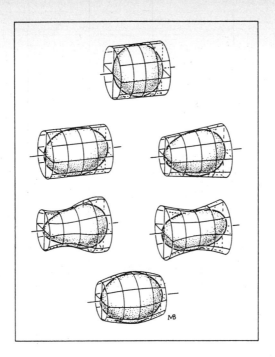

Fig. 2.4.1 Co-ordinate transforms of the x, y plane, when rotated about the x-axis generate transformed spaces. The transformed sphere generates a variety of egg shapes.

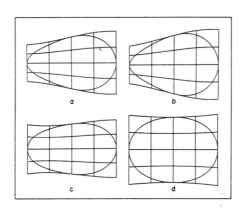

Fig. 2.4.2 Co-ordinate transformations for: (a) $f(X) = 0.56 + 0.2X - 0.02X^2 - 0.07X^3$ (Common Murre), (b) $f(X) = 0.63 + 0.24X - 0.05X^2 - 0.07X^3$ (Brunrich's Murre), (c) $f(X) = 0.54 + 0.1X + 0.04X^2 - 0.06X^3$ (Red Throated Loon), (d) $f(X) = 0.7 + 0.01X + 0.05X^2$ (Cassovary).

Deriving the transformation : We may derive the transformation
necessary to yield a given egg profile by reversing the formula for
the egg shape

$$f(X) = \frac{y}{\sqrt{a^2 - x^2}}$$

f(X) thus derived may now be approximated by a polynomial of a
given order. Inspection of plots of f(x) for various eggs (fig.
2.4.3) suggests the appropriate order of polynomial. By approximating the transformation function f by polynomials of particular
orders we produce a quantification of the shape of the egg (the n +
1 coefficients of our nth order polynomial comprise the quantitative data). This is equivalent to the classification due to
Preston (1953). The transformed coordinate approach, however is
not only more easy to visualise, but also applicable to other systems.

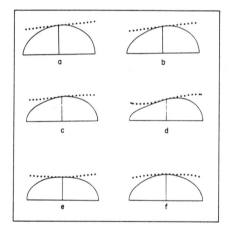

Fig. 2.4.3 Approximations to the function f(X) derived from formula
(4) for (a) the thrush, (b) the common term, (c) an ab-
normally shaped hen's egg, (d) the common guillemot, (e)
the kiwi and (f) the emu. (a) and (b) yield approximately linear f, (e) and (f) quadratic and (c) and (d)
cubic.

From equations of the above form, the average curvature of the egg
at any point may be derived.

For a surface of revolution
$$S = \{(x, y, z) : \sqrt{y^2 + z^2} = r(x)\}$$

The average curvature is

$$H = \frac{(1 + (\frac{dr}{dx})^2 - r\frac{d^2r}{dx^2})}{2r(1 + (\frac{dr}{dx})^2)^{\frac{3}{2}}}$$

(2,4,10)

if $r(x) = f(X) \sqrt{1 - X^2}$ $[X = \frac{x}{a}]$

then

$$\frac{dr}{dx} = \frac{(1 - X^2)\frac{df}{dX} - Xf}{a\sqrt{1 - X^2}}$$

(2.4.11)

$$\frac{d^2r}{dx^2} = \frac{(1 - X^2)\frac{d^2f}{dX^2} - 2X(1 - X^2)\frac{df}{dX} - f}{a^2(1 - X^2)^{\frac{3}{2}}}$$

(2.4.12)

$\frac{1}{H}$ may be derived by substituting 2.4.11 and 2.4.12 in 2.4.10

Spline Model of Egg Geometry

The second method of obtaining an analytic representation of the egg's outline is rather less elegant, but more generally applicable. It involves the acquisition of direct digital approximation to the surface curvature at points on the outline of the egg. A prerequisite to such digital approximation is a knowledge of the positon of the egg's axis of symmetry. We describe the procedure used:

The starting point for our analysis is a photograph of the egg under investigation. The analysis takes the following form:

(a   The outline of the egg is digitised from a photograph using a magnetic graphics tablet. Preliminary analysis filters out overlap of the beginning and end of the digitised curve and 'joins up the ends'.

(b)   Parametric cubic splines are fitted to the points to give an analytic description of the egg's outline.

(c) The best fit to an axis of symmetry for the spline curve is approximated.

(d) Average curvature H of the surface of revolution about this axis is evaluated digitally at each of the original data points, and a Cubic spline curve fit to 1/H. This curve is then plotted over the outline of the egg from b above.

A spline curve fitted to 1/H(x) and plotted above the egg outline (X(t), Y(t)). The tension in the wall of the oviduct is

$$T_W(x) = P/H(x) - T_O$$

The graph of 1/H(x) is therefore in effect a graph of the tension in the wall of the oviduct. Figure 2.4.4 shows different shaped eggs in a variety of species, and the oviduct tensions which generate these shapes.

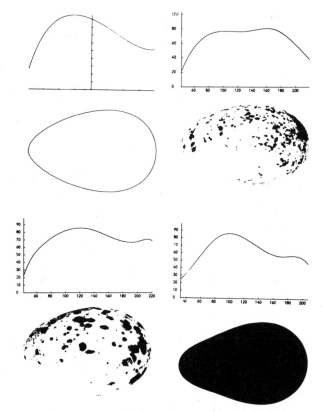

Figure 2.4.4. Graphs of 1/H measured from (a) a standard ovoid (b) a common gull's egg (c) a heming gull egg (d) a guillemot egg.

Discussion

We pick up here the strands of argument from this example which are felt to be of importance to the major themes of this monograph.

Firstly, of peripheral interest, is the use of D'Arcy Thomson's co-ordinate transforms to indicate an analytical model for the shape of the eggs' shells. The economy of this technique suggests it as a general method of shape quantification. Shape descriptors play an important role in many areas of quantitative biology, and com-puterised measuring techniques give access to greater quantities of shape information. The type of shape descriptors currently used - for example perimeter/area ratio, max diameter/min diameter ratio - are both crude and difficult to interpret when applied to complex shapes. The transformed coordinate technique allows a flexible level of complexity of quantification as approximate transforma-tions of greater or lesser degrees of sophistication may be used. By using a complex 'base structure' simple but meaningful quantifi-cations of the shape of homologous structures may be made.

The key elements of this analysis are the following:-

(i)   a suitable base structure is set. In our case the circle.

(ii) a family of allowed transformations is decided upon, with a suitable number of parameters. The values taken by these parameters, for the best fit transformation, are then our shape quantifiers.

In the example considered in this paper the parameters k, c, d, e for the best fit cubic transformation characterise the shape of the egg. As defined, these parameters are scale invariant and there-fore constitute true shape descriptors. They are in suitable form to apply some form of discriminatory analysis, and could therefore form the basis of an egg-shape taxonomy.

All forms of quantitative image analysis either performed by squared paper and ruler or by sophisticated modern equipment have

as their end result a set of real number parameters purporting to
echo some real life property of the object under study. Statistical analysis of these parameters is then used to make a statement
about the probable validity of some hypothesis. D'Arcy Thomson's
coordinate transformations provide a useful method of providing
such image description parameter.

Of more direct interest to the development of this thesis are the
two approaches to geometrical surface representation attempted
above. On the one hand a simple analytic model of the surface
yielded results which amply depicted the qualitative characteristics of the system. This simple model was appropriate in the
analysis of birds' eggs, which are regular in shape.

The second approach, that of splining, yields a less tractable geometry, but is applicable to less regular shapes. In models of various biological phenomena, we shall see repeated this duality of
modelling strategies: on the one hand a mathematically appealing
model which represents only the main features of the biological
surface, on the other hand a mathematically less attractive model
which fits the biology more exactly.

The feature of the egg model of central interest to this thesis is
that the surface geometry of the egg results directly from the physical pressures exerted on it during its formation. Analysis of
the geometry therefore yields insight into those physical processes.

2.5 The Folding Pattern of the Cerebral Cortex

The relationship between the pattern of folding of the mammalian
cerebral cortex and the functional and anatomical structure of the
brain as a whole has long been an object of controversy amongst comparative neuroanatomists. In this case study we shall focus on the
relationship between the folding pattern and the surface geometry
of the brain. Specifically, we shall investigate the hypothesis
that folding tends to follow lines of minimal curvature on the
brain's surface.

Two mechanical models of the process of cortical folding have been published. Le Gros Clark (1945) suggests a mixture of extrinsic factors causing sulci to develop perpendicular to postulated lines of 'growth stress', and intrinsic factors causing sulci to develop either at the join between areas of cortex with different mechanical properties ('limiting sulci'), or at the centre of such an area ('axial sulci'). Thus the general trend or direction of the folding is determined in his model by the geometry of the growth process, whereas the specific sites of folding are determined by the cellular constitution of the cortex. Richman, Stewart, Hutchinson and Caviness (1975) propose a mechanical model for the development of tertiary convolutions in the human cortex, driven by stresses created by differential elasticity between an outer stratum (layers I, II, III) and an inner stratum (layers IV, V, VI). From estimates of the parameters: the Young's Modulus of each of the strata and of the core material, and the thickness of the two strata, this model is able to predict the wavelength of folding. With suitable values for these parameters, the model reflects the various convolutional patterns observed in normal, microgyric and lissencephalic human brains. In effect a link is elicited between the microstructure of the cortex, as embodied in the Young's Moduli and thickness of the strata, and the folding pattern. in this case study we shall examine the other end of the problem and elaborate on the relationship, implicit in Le Gros Clark's model, between the geometry of the brain in the large and the folding pattern.

It is necessary to clearly define what is meant here by the folding pattern. Mature cortical folds are narrow slit-like fissures and define linear markings on the surface of the brain. The pattern formed by these markings, and in particular their direction, we refer to as the folding pattern. Given the surface geometry of a brain, we desire a field of directions on that surface; this field specifying the direction in which folding should occur. We do not consider the many issues which determine whether a fold should occur in the first place.

Cortical Folding

The cerebral hemispheres of all vertebrates are initially smooth.
In some animals the cerebral cortex, which comprises a surface
layer of the cerebral hemispheres, becomes folded. The neurons
which will make up the adult cortex are produced in a relatively
short period during prenatal development. They are derived from a
precursor population which lines the ventricle at the interior of
the hemisphere. The newly-born neurons migrate to their eventual
surface position guided by a system of radial fibres which connect
the central production site with the periphery of the cerebral
hemispheres. After neuron production has finished, smooth brains
expand retaining approximately the same shape as the embryonic
form. Folded brains exhibit a different behaviour.

> At the time when cortical neurons have largely completed
> their proliferation and migration to the surface of the
> hemispheres, the immature cortex is still relatively
> smooth. Convolutions develop gradually during the late
> fetal and early postnatal periods. The expansion of sur-
> face area of the cortex during this period is probably due
> more to an increase in cell size than cell number. Thus
> the growth rates of different cortical regions should be
> relatively similar, assuming that cortical thickness and
> cell density do not vary radically throughout the hem-
> isphere." (Van Essen and Maunsell 1980)

A geometric folding model

There is considerable growth during the period of folding. However
a distinction must be made between uniform growth, which will increase the size of a surface but not affect its intrinsic geometry
(or 'shape') and differential growth, which may affect both. Van
Essen and Maunsell (1980) define two processes to account for cortical convolutions: folding and change of intrinsic curvature. Folding is that part of the shape transformation which may be achieved
without differential growth. An example of pure folding is a sheet
of newspaper crumpled into a ball. Change in intrinsic curvature

is any shape transformation which requires differential growth. In our idealised model, we shall assume that growth is uniform. Therefore the cortical convolutions must be formed by pure 'folding'. As uniform growth does not influence the geometry of the surface, it will henceforth be ignored and our model will consider brains changing in shape but not in size.

The radial organisation of the cortex is important both during its development and during its functional life (Rakic 1981). A system of radial fibres connects the cortex with the subcortical tissue. Initially these are fibres which act as guides to migrating neurons. Later other fibres connect cortical neurons to subcortical fibre tracts. On a purely mechanical level, however, these radial fibres will act against any transverse motion or slipping of the cortex over the subcortical tissue during folding. We embody this observation into our model as a principle of minimal radial distortion. During the process of folding we require as little gross slipping of the cortex over the subcortical tissue as possible; hence the least possible disruption of cortical/subcortical fibrous connections.

We now assert that a cortex developing under the combined restraints of uniform growth and minimal radial distortion will tend to fold along lines of minimal curvature. It was observed above that folding starts with dimple formation. Looking at a small region of convex surface local to a point A, a dimple may be made by pushing in a portion of the surface (fig. 2.5.1a). This elementary folding operation involves no dislocation of surface material outside the dimple, and little distortion inside. To a first approximation, the figure formed by the perimeter of the dimple is an ellipse Struik (1950) whose long axis is parallel to the direction of minimal curvature at A, and whose short axis is parallel to the direction of maximal curvature at A.

In the model the sides of the dimple are now pinched in to form a narrow slit-like fissure characteristic of the mature cortical fold. Minimal transverse dislocation of cortical tissue is attained if the dimple is pinched so that the fold is aligned along the long axis of the ellipse (fig. 2.5.1b). We therefore assert that folding will tend to occur along lines of minimal curvature on the cortical surface.

50

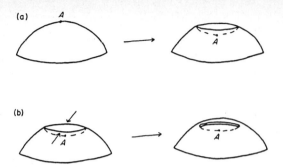

Fig. 2.5.1 A hypothetical fold is produced at an elliptical point A of a surface. (a) A dimple is formed by reflecting through a plane parallel to the tangent plane at A. (b) The dimple is squeezed along its short axis to form a narrow slit.

In order to analyse the patterns of minimal curvature on a brain, it is necessary to have a mathematical model of its surface geometry. Geometrically simple models, however, are of interest. Although the model shape is not a precise analogue of that of the brain under study, such models, because of their mathematical simplicity, may be easily analysed. They also require rather simple measurements, which may be taken from 2dimensional pictures of the brain. Here we first model the cerebral surface as radially symmetric about an axis parallel to its mid-line. The model surface is then entirely characterised by a single 2-dimensional view; we take the outline afforded by a dorsal picture of the brain. The axisymmetric model is applied to a variety of brains, and is capable of picking out major trends to longitudinal or transverse folding. A second model, applied to the canid brain, approximates the cerebral surface by a segment of triaxial ellipsoid; the required parameters - the lengths of the three semi-axes - are measured from dorsal and lateral views of the brain. The lines of minimal curvature on this ellipsoid follow quite closely the pattern of folding observed on the canid brain.

Axisymmetric model

The lines of principal curvature on an axisymmetric surface are the lines on the surfaces parallel to and perpendicular to the axis of symmetry, known respectively as meridians and parallels. If the curvature of the meridian at a given point is less than the normal curvature in the perpendicular direction, then the meridian is the line of minimal curvature, and by our hypothesis folding should be longitudinal. Otherwise the parallel is the line of minimal curvature, and folding should be transverse.

The shape of the axisymmetric model is determined from a single 2-dimensional view of the brain. Figure 2.5.2 shows the lines of minimal curvature on axisymmetric models of brains of a variety of species. The process for constructing the models is described in figure 2.5.3. The general trend which emerges is transverse folding in the wider central regions of the cortex, and longitudinal folding in the tapered front and rear. The proportion of transverse to longitudinal folding depends of the shape of the brain. The short wide echidna brain (a) is largely transversely folded, while the relatively longer thinner capybara brain (c) has mainly longitudinal folds. The 25 week human embryonic brain (d) exhibits a similar regime of folding, longitudinal front and back, transverse in the middle. The axisymmetric model has the virtue of being simple to apply, picks out longitudinal versus transverse folding trends, but is unable to produce more complicated folding patterns. For this we need a geometrically richer model, and turn to the simplest truly three dimensional closed surface: the ellipsoid.

Ellipsoid model

The lines of principal curvature of an ellipsoid, when projected onto a plane perpendicular to its short axis, consist of a system of co-axial ellipses and of portions of a system of hyperbolae having the same axes (figure 2.5.4). There are four umbilics on the surface. The lines of minimal curvature of the ellipsoid projected in this manner are the elliptical curvature lines and the long axis between the two umbilics.

The shape of triaxial ellipsoid is specified by three linear measurements: the lengths of the three perpendicular axes. To model a portion of brain surface as a portion of triaxial ellipsoid, then, it is necessary to have two perpendicular views of the brain from which to measure these axes. For the canid brain, axes were measured from dorsal and lateral views published in Radinsky

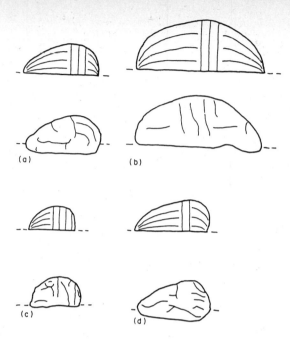

Figure 2.5.2 Dorsal views of the brains of (a) macropus (b) 26 week
human embryo (c) echidna (d) capybara. (a), (c), (d)
after Ariens Kappers (1936) (b) after Chi (1977).
Above each is an axisymmetric model constructed in the
way depicted in Fig. 2.5.3. Regions on the models
with lines marked perpendicular to the axis represent
regions where minimal curvature is transverse. Regions with lines marked running front to back have
longitudinal lines of minimal curvature.

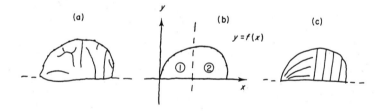

Figure 2.5.3 Construction of an axisymmetric model. (a) At regular
intervals along the middle of the brain, the width of
the brain is measured from a dorsal view. (b) A curve
$y = f(x)$ is fit through these points by computer. Now
the surface formed by rotating this curve about the
x-axis is the three-dimensional model of the brain geometry. The principal curvatures are $k_1 = f''/(1 + f'^2)^{3/2}$
in the longitudinal direction and $k_2 = 1/f\sqrt{1 + (f')^2}$
in the transverse. Where $k_1 < k_2$ then folding is
deemed to be longitudinal (area 1); otherwise folding
is transverse (area 2). (c) These areas are represented schematically by longitudinal and transverse
lines on the model.

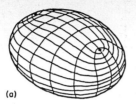 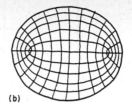

(a)   (b)

Fig. 2.5.4   (a) Lines of principal curvature on a triaxial ellip-
              soid, (b) these lines projected onto the plane perpend-
              icular to the short axis of the ellipsoid. The lines of
              principal curvature on an ellipsoid with semi axis
              lengths a, b, c where a > b > c, when projected onto a
              plane perpendicular to the short axis are coaxial el-
              lipses and hyperbolae with axis lengths a' and b' such
              that:
              a'²(a² - c²)/a²(a² - b²) + b'²(b² - c²)/b²(b² - a²) = 1
              (Salmon 1912).

(1973b). A projection of the ellipsoid, with its attendant lines
of minimal curvature, corresponding to a lateral view of the brain
is then produced (fig. 2.5.5). The correspondence between these
lines of minimal curvature and the folds on the canid cortex is
close. The folds form a system of coaxial semi-ellipses similar to
the lines of minimal curvature on the ellipsoid model.

The above pattern of minimal curvatures remains structurally stable
so long as the axis perpendicular to the lateral plane is the short
axis of the ellipsoid. The change in form if the perpendicular
axis is lengthened to equal and exceed the middle axis is illustrated in figure 2.5.5. When the two axes are equal, we revert to
the axisymmetric case, with longitudinal folding. When the axis is
further increased, projections of the lines of minimal curvature
comprise a system of elliptical segments which do not join. This
may be seen to echo the longitudinal folding pattern observed in
the prosimian galago crassiscaudatus (fig. 2.5.5). The folding pattern of the simian primates, complicated by increased operculation
of the sylvan fissure, has its roots in this parallel prosimian
folding pattern. The transition from carnivore to primate brain
folding is modelled by this flip from one system of minimal curvatures to the other as lateral dimension exceeds the vertical in the
prosimian.

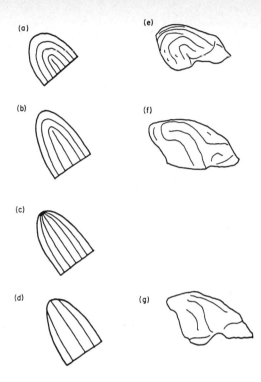

Figure 2.5.5   Ellipsoid brain models: (e) the canid Lycaon pictus
and the prosimians, (f) Indri indri and (g) Galago
crassicaudatus.   (a), (b) and (d) are side views of
ellipsoids whose dimensions correspond to those of
the frontal portions of the brains.   These dimensions were measured from lateral and dorsal views
published in Radinsky (1973, 1968).   In (a) and (b)
the axis perpendicular to the page is the short
axis.   In (d) it is the middle axis.   (c) is an
intermediate stage where the axis perpendicular to
the page is equal to the shorter axis on the page.
Lines of minimum curvature, calculated as described
in Fig. 2.5.3 are drawn on these ellipsoids.

Structural stability

The ellipsoid model is capable of depicting the sort of relationship which may hold between the geometry of the brain and the
stability of the folding pattern.   If there is a significant difference between the lengths of the three axes, the pattern of lines
of minimal curvature is stable with respect to small variations in
these lengths.   If, however, the lengths are similar, that is the
surface is close to spherical, then small variations may drastic-
ally alter the pattern of the lines of minimal curvature (fig.
2.5.6).   In a hypothetical species whose brains were proper ellipsoids, slight variations in the geometry of the brain between

individuals would have no great effect on the pattern of the folding (structurally stable). On the other hand, a species with a
spherical brain would experience drastic differences between individual folding patterns in response to minor differences in individual brain geometries (structurally unstable).

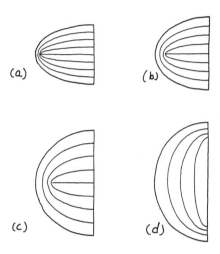

Figure 2.5.6   A small change in the axes for an asymmetric ellip-
                soid (a) → (b) causes little change in the pattern
                of minimal curvatures. Small changes in the length
                of axes for a close to symmetric ellipsoid (c) → (d)
                can cause a qualitative change in the pattern of
                minimal curvatures.

In an analogous way, the relationship between the geometry of the
real cortex and the folding pattern suggests that some species
should have stable folding patterns from specimen to specimen,
while others should experiences considerable intraspecies variation. This phenomenon has been observed and commented upon. More-
over, the geometry of a species may yield unstable folding in a
particular region, perhaps a spheroidal region, and stable folding
in another region, perhaps ellipsoidal. This would induce high
inter-animal variation in a restricted region of the cortex, which
has been observed (fig. 2.5.7).

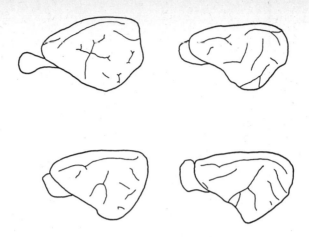

Fig. 2.5.7   Capybara brains exhibit considerable inter-animal
               variation in folding pattern.

Discussion

In this case study, we have presented qualitative evidence for a relation between the external pattern of folding on a simple folded
cortex and the geometry of the embryonic brain. Such a relation is
interesting for the light it may throw on the connection between
neuron production and abnormal folding patterns; also for the insight it could provide to the phylogenetic importance of changing
sulcal patterns and the significance of sulci as functional landmarks.

Two mechanical models of the process of cortical folding have been
published. Le Gros Clark (1945) suggests a mixture of extrinsic
factors causing sulci to develop perpendicular to postulated lines
of 'growth stress', and intrinsic factors causing sulci to develop
either at the join between areas of cortex with different mechanical properties ('limiting sulci'), or at the centre of such an area
('axial sulci'). Thus the general trend or direction of the folding is determined in his model by the geometry of the growth process, whereas the specific sites of folding are determined by the
cellular constitution of the cortex. Richman, Stewart, Hutchinson

and Caviness (1975) propose a mechanical model for the development
of tertiary convolutions in the human cortex, driven by stresses
created by differential elasticity between an outer stratum (layers
I, II, III) and an inner stratum (layers IV, V, VI). This model is
able to predict the wavelength of folding from estimates of the
elasticity of each of the strata and of the core material, and the
thickness of the two strata. With suitable values for these parameters, the model reflects the various convolutional patterns observed in normal, microgyric and lissencephalic human brains. In
effect a link is elicited between the microstructure of the cortex,
as embodied in the Young's Moduli and thickness of the strata, and
the folding pattern. In this study we have examined the other end
of the problem and elaborate on the relationship, implicit in Le
Gros Clark's model, between the geometry of the brain in the large
and the folding pattern.

The geometry of a biological surface is closely related to the
growth regime which produced the surface. The cortical surface
first grows as a result of neuron production, and then during the
folding process, as a result of myelination and cell growth concomitant with differentiation. Hence a link is effected between
the pattern of neuron production and the folding patterns on the
adult brain, via the geometry of the embryonic, post-production,
pre-folding, cortex. Localised deficiencies in neuron production,
either experimentally induced, or as a result of developmental dis-
order, would distort the geometry of the embryonic brain, which distortion would manifest itself as an abnormal folding pattern in the
adult. Richman et al. (1975) and Evrard, Caviness, Prato-Vinas and
Lyon (1978) seek a link between cell production deficiencies and abnormal depth and wavelength of folding via the pathological cytoarchitecture of the cortex, and a mechanical model. Here we have
linked cell production with the overall folding pattern through the
geometry of the embryonic brain.

The surfaces of even smooth brains are geometrically rather complex. In this case study, we have used two grossly simplified
models of the geometry. The advantage of these models was that
they could be constructed from two-dimensional pictures of the
brain. A more sophisticated analysis of the relationship between
the geometry of the brain and the folding pattern requires a

three-dimensional digitisation of the prefolded brain, and is the subject of a later chapter.

2.6 Surface Curvatures of the Cerebral Cortex

In the previous example, the geometry of folding in the cerebral cortex was related to the overall geometry of the brain via the curvature of the cortical surface. In this case study we consider the change in the intrinsic geometry of the surface of the brain during folding. In the model of 2.5, growth was assumed to be uniform and therefore no change in intrinsic geometry was provided for. In this section, we drop the assumption of uniform growth and develop tools to analyse the changes in the surface geometry of the brain during the process of folding.

It was noted above that the cerebral cortex may usefully be regarded as a surface phenomenon. Two further characteristics of the cortex should be borne in mind in the ensuing discussion. On the one hand, the cortex is remarkably uniform in its physical structure; on the other hand there is evidence to suggest that some distinct functional areas of the cortex tend to align themselves with the folding pattern of the brain. These two observations lend weight to two contending models of brain folding. The first model, supported by the first observation, imposes folding on a uniformly growing cortex. These are the assumptions of section 2.4 above. The antithesis is a model where folding is caused by the differential growth of specific areas of the brain, possibly in conjunction with some functional specialisation. Assuming that the folding of a real cortex is a synthesis of the two extreme models, we examine the role of surface curvatures as parameters of the synthesis.

Decomposition of shape transforms

Three distinct types of geometrical transformations are combined in different proportions in each of these models.

(i)   <u>Dilatation</u>: Dilatation represents pure 'scaling up' where the shape of the surface is unchanged, but its size is enlarged (or reduced). If we took a flat square surface (say a square sheet of paper) and dilated it, the result would be a flat square, larger or smaller than the original by the 'scale factor' of the dilatation. A dilatation of scale factor 2 would be double the length and breadth of the sheet. If we dilated a spherical surface, the result would be a larger (or smaller) sphere. In general size will be of less interest in our modelling than shape. Hence dilatations will be in general 'factored out', or ignored in our models.

(ii)   <u>Isometry</u>: An isometry is a transformation which is achieved by bending a surface without stretching or tearing it. An isometric transformation involves no growth of the surface and all distances, as long as they are measured on the surface, remain the same. In the context of the cerebral cortex, an isometry can be described as 'pure folding' (van Essen and Maunsell, 1980). Examples of surface isometry are folding a flat sheet to form a cylinder, or poking a dimple into a sphere (2.5 above).

(iii)   <u>Differential Growth</u>: This category includes any transformation which requires non-uniform stretching or distortion of the surface. This type of transformation alters the intrinsic geometry of the surface in a non-uniform way. An example of differential growth is the truncated sphere to sphere model of 2.5.2. The process required to make a flat map of the earth's surface is a further example of this type of transformation.

In the nomenclature of van Essen and Maunsell the contrast between transformation (ii) and (iii) is between 'folding' and 'intrinsic curvature'. A uniform growth model for cortical folding admits dilation and isometry only. A differential growth model admits all types of transformation.

From a biological standpoint, the importance of decomposing a transformation in this way lies in the fact that different types of growth and growth control are associated with each fundamental type of transformation.

Dilatation can be achieved by uniform growth. Uniform growth is a widespread biological phenomenon and of little interest in itself. We shall thus generally 'factor out' uniform growth by ignoring scale and concentrating on shape in the following.

Isometric transformation, as noted above, involves no change in the intrinsic geometry of a surface. Such a transformation may not then be caused by factors internal to the surface but must be due to the influence of external forces.

It should be noted at this point that the mathematical surfaces referred to are 2-dimensional entities with no depth. On the other hand a biological surface such as the cerebral cortex has depth. One model of cortical folding (Richman et al 1975) is driven by inhomogeneities in the elastic properties of the material at different depths in the cortex. Although such influences are internal to the cortex, their effect is perpendicular to it and mathematically they must be described as 'external influences'. An external influence in a biological setting is therefore one whose line of action is perpendicular (normal) to the surface. An internal influence is one which acts in a direction tangential to the surface.

Differential growth is that part of a surface transformation which requires a regime of different local growth rates. Both intrinsic and extrinsic factors may be active in generating the resultant shape transformation.

Any shape transformation may be described by a differential growth; in this essay we shall be interested in the extent to which differential growth needs to be involved to generate the shape transformation. We seek to distinguish between shape transformations which can be generated by 'uniform growth + isometry' ('similarities' in the sequel) and shape transformations which require differential growth. In the latter case we shall try to quantify the differential growth element in the transformation. This we can regard as a measure of the change in intrinsic geometry of the surface.

Surface Curvatures as Parameters of Growth

The different surface curvatures are connected with different elements of this isometry/non-isometry, extrinsic/intrinsic balance.
They are therefore useful parameters of the cmposition of a shape
transform. Gaussian Curvature, $K = K_{max} . K_{min}$ is invariant
under isometry. K has dimensions length $^{-2}$, dilatation would
thus cause K to vary inversely with the square of the scale factor.
A model of cortical development as uniform growth with folding
superimposed would thus result in a net decrease in K. Average
curvature on the other hand may be profoundly affected by isometric
transformations. A flat sheet of paper may be rolled into a cylinder of any radius without tearing or stretching it. The average
curvature of the paper, originally 0 is now $1/2r$. We see that
changes in average curvature may reflect purely extrinsic changes
in a surface. However changes in intrinsic geometry of the surface
will also result in a change in average curvature. For example a
flat sheet growing into a sphere of radius undergoes a change in
average curvature from 0 to $1/r$.

The main interest of van Essen and Maunsell is in making flat maps
of folded brains. They find that they are able to 'unfold' a cortex and flatten it with relatively little distortion. They therefore speculate that much of the shape transformation between smooth
and folded cortex is 'pure folding', and they link this with a uniform growth model of cortical maturation. In Chapters 4 and 5 we
will develop a technique to measure the curvatures K, H, and
$H^2 - K$ directly. This will enable us to follow experimentally
the actual shape transformation of a folding ferret brain and pronounce on the validity of the above authors' speculations.

2.7 Coda

This chapter consisted of five separate case studies where surface
geometry has played a role in the modelling of a biological phenomenon. On a technical mathematical level, we have introduced the
vocabulary of elementary differential geometry: the first and
second fundamental forms, surface curvature, Gauss's theorem. On a

more fundamental level, we wish to summarise the major themes underlying our approach to these case studies. It is these themes which will be reintroduced in the following chapters.

A strategy for selecting the appropriate geometric model for a biological system, when there are several models available has consistently been to select for minimum complexity. In the root growth and cerebral vesicle models this meant demanding isotropy and axisymmetry of the growth function. Simplicity in the egg model meant representing the egg-shell membrane as uniform and isotropic and the external pressure of the oviduct static. The assumption of uniform growth in the case study on the geometry of cortical folding is a further example of this 'economy of complexity' principle.

In general, the aim of mathematical modelling is to examine an analogue to a real system operating under some simplifying assumptions. A system is its own best analogue so some sort of selection for simplicity is essential. A principle which states that the simplest model which retains the particular traits of the system which are currently of interest may therefore claim to be a general guide to the selection of mathematical models.

In harmony with the general requirement for simplicity in models, two approaches to expressing the geometry of a biological surface emerge from the above examples. The first approach is to use a simple mathematical surface which very loosely approximates the shape of the biological surface. This approach is exemplified in the hemispheric root tip model, the disc to truncated sphere model for cerebral vesicle formation, the linear deformation of a sphere model for the shape of a bird's egg, the axisymmetric and ellipsoid models for the geometry of the brain. Where the former approach does not model the biological surface in sufficient detail, a numerical rather than analytic mathematical model is sought. An example of this type of model is the spline model for the shape of the egg.

In all the above case studies, the geometry of a biological surface shed light on the intrinsic and extrinsic factors influencing that geometry. In the root tip and vesicle models it was the intrinsic differential growth of the tissue which was of interest, in the egg model it was the extrinsic effect of the pressure of the oviduct on the egg shell. The model which postulates the brain folding along lines of minimal curvature is presenting a coherent theory connecting brain shape to folding pattern while assuming purely extrinsic factors at work in an otherwise uniform cortex. The purpose of introducing the different measures of surface curvature in section 2.6 was to provide parameters for the extrinsic and intrinsic nature of surface shape change: to distinguish between uniform growth + isometry (indicative of purely external influences) and differential growth (internal influence). The biological significance of the distinction between extrinsic and intrinsic factors at work in the cerebral cortex will be examined in greater depth in chapter 4.

CHAPTER 3

MINIMUM DIRICHLET INTEGRAL OF GROWTH RATE AS
A METRIC FOR INTRINSIC SHAPE DIFFERENCE

3.1 Introduction

In this chapter, a general theoretical framework for constructing
models of biological surfaces is put forward. The examples of the
previous chapter may be regarded as introducing the vocabulary for
the following development. In particular, the geometric strategy
may be seen as a generalisation of the approach used in sections
2.2 and 2.3 to model tip growth and mouse cerebral vesicle development.

Some preamble is perhaps appropriate here on the place of mathematical modelling in biological science. Biology is a complex field in
which there is currently little hope of some unifying mathematical
simplification, such as that afforded to celestial physics by New-
tonian mechanics. The range of biological phenomena is too diverse
for their essential nature to be encapsulated in some single mathematical formulation. We cannot conclude, however, that all mathematical modelling in biology is futile; individual problems may be
advantageously represented by mathematical models. Several examples of such models have been discussed in previous chapters. Here
we are interested in the philosophy behind the modelling process.

The area of science where mathematical modelling has achieved its
most spectacular successes is in physics. A property of mathematical physics is that its models are self-contained, they do not
invoke extraneous fields of knowledge; indeed their precepts are
designated 'physical laws'. This is at variance with the approach
taken in many classes of models in mathematical biology, which
recast biological problems in physical terms and then apply the
well-developed mathematics of physics. Examples of such an approach include the mechanical brain folding model of Richman et al.
(1975), fluid dynamical models of blood flow, work on the dynamics

of animal locomotion. The value of such models is not in dispute, and they do serve to describe one aspect of these biological phenomena. We should however note another group of models in mathematical biology which do not invoke the physical sciences, but which have their roots wholly in biology. Examples of this type of model include the Volterra-Lotka predator-prey relationship, the Hodgkin-Huxley nerve transmission equations, evolutionary game theory. These models use their own essentially biological mathematics, without explicit dependence on the mathematics of physics. There is no need to appeal to the physical sciences to claim credibility for a mathematical model in biology. If a self contained mathematical framework can be constructed, which is consistent with an adequate subset of the biological facts, then this may be a legitimate model.

We shall attempt in this chapter to give a self-consistent mathematical framework for treating biological surface growth. Its principles, like physical laws, we shall not attempt to justify from outside biology. On the other hand, although physical laws need not be justified, the discovery of a particular set of useful principles normally follows a train of intuitive reasoning. In this way, the Hodgkin-Huxley equations for electrical transmission in nerve fibres, while they can be regarded as empirical equations, may also be intuitively 'derived' using an argument involving the presence of sodium and potassium channels, and blocking molecules (Jones & Sleeman 1983).

In this chapter, we shall alternate between two standpoints: from one standpoint our model is viewed purely as a mathematical entity, and judged on its internal consistency and usefulness in characterising some properties of certain biological systems. From another standpoint, the mathematics may be derived from some apparently more elementary properties of the biological structure which is being modelled. In our case these 'more elementary properties' are rather vague, and we are probably on firmer ground adopting the former standpoint. The vagueness of the premises for our intuitive derivation is not, however, unique to this problem and is in fact the rule rather than the exception in models of physical systems. We shall not be deterred by these doubts and shall give in the following both an intuitive derivation and a straight definition of our methodology.

In the root tip model of 2.2, axisymmetry and isotropy were taken
as foundations on which to build a mathematical model for biological surface growth. Both these principles were chosen for the
economy with wich they described the physical process of growth.
This economy could be seen as a property either of the biological
system or merely of the mathematical model.

Bookstein (1978) discussing Green's (1965) work on Nitella tip
growth comments,

> "Such a strategy, despite its elegance, cannot
> be expected to generalise to systems lacking the
> peculiar symmetries of the organ, radial sym-
> metry and invariance of form over time, as the
> necessary differential equations can no longer
> be produced."

Here as we are satisfied with generating a discrete time model, invariance of form over time is not essential, we require only a knowledge of the initial and final forms. Abandoning radial symmetry,
however, is more serious. There are in general an infinite number
of mappings between two surfaces which correspond to istropic
growth; in the absence of symmetry, it is necessary to find a
replacement principle to guide the choice of the appropriate
mapping. The principle we shall use is the minimisation of the
Dirichlet integral of the average growth rate over the initial
surface.

We consider two mathematical surfaces S and T representing two
stages in some biological process. We are interested in the
patterns of growth which would generate T from S. Note that the
term 'growth' here and in the sequel is used to include both expan-
sion and contraction, although the latter goes against everyday
usage of the term. A large balloon may 'grow' into a small one by
contracting when the air is released. For the present we shall
restrict the growth to being isotropic, and shall assume that the
mathematical surfaces S and T admit isotropic mapping, that is S
and T are 'conformally equivalent'. Conditions for conformal
equivalence will be discussed below.

Isotropy implies that growth is determined by a field of scalar growth factors $\lambda(s)$ defined on S such that the first fundamental forms of corresponding points on S and T are in the ratio λ^2

i.e., $dt^2 = \lambda^2 ds^2$.

The average rate of growth $\mu - \log \lambda$ associated with the growth factor λ defines a growth potential field on the surface S.

Define

$$D[\lambda] = \iint_S (\nabla \log \lambda)^2 \qquad\qquad (4.2.1)$$

$D[\lambda]$ is the Dirichlet integral of $\log\lambda$ over S and is a measure of the smoothness of the potential μ. We argue that the smoother the growth function, the simpler the control mechanism necessary to run it and the less 'energy of control' required. Hence, we assert, the conformal map with minimal $D[\lambda]$ is the simplest such mapping, and therefore, for the modeller's purposes, the best.

An alternative way of viewing this hypothesis is to assume a general trend towards continuity of cellular experience in biological tissue. The 'smoothest possible mapping' hypothesis emerges naturally from a local averaging rule of the type proposed by Goodwin (1977).

3.2 Isotropic and Anisotropic Biological Growth

Before analysing the properties of the minimum Dirichlet integral model introduced in the previous section, it is worthwhile for us to discuss the domain of validity, in nature, of the assumptions underpinning the model. In particular, by adopting isotropy as a simplifying mathematical assumption, we necessarily restrict the range of biological systems for which our modelling strategy is

applicable to those which do not exhibit anisotropy of the growth
process. In this section, we shall look at the occurrence of isotropic and anisotropic surface growth in biology and discuss the
biological reasoning behind the adoption of isotropy as a null
hypothesis.

Isotropy is a property which expresses a lack of directional preference of growth at the local level. The large scale geometrical
change resulting from istropic growth can, however, exhibit direc-
tionality. In the example of section 2.2 the growth of a plant's
stalk, which is unidirectional along its axis, is achieved by isotropic growth at the tip of the stalk. In fact any surface transformation (subject to technical mathematical restrictions discussed
below) can be achieved by isotropic growth. To establish whether
isotropy is a sensible model for a particular biological system,
one needs either to examine the mechanisms responsible for the
growth, and determine whether a directional preference is present,
or to empirically derive evidence of isotropy from experimental
analysis of the small scale growth itself.

Experimental attempts to ascertian isotropy or anisotropy in developing plant walls have involved measuring the distortion induced
on either real or hypothetical circles marked on the growing surface. Green (1969), studying tip growth in fungi, claims that such
systems are largely isotopic, Nitella however being an exception.
His experimental technique involves physically drawing circles on
the developing cell wall. An obvious constraint on this procedure
is that the dimensions of the circle must be small with respect ot
variations in the growth rate; otherwise such variations in a
genuinely isotropic tissue may be misconstrued as indications of
anisotropy. Erickson (1966) finds that leaf growth in Xanthius is
"largely isotropic, though the margins are somewhat anisotropic."
His experimental method is to trace the positions on a growing leaf
of a number of points, identified by the venation pattern. He then
interpolates a velocity field numerically, and analysis of the
divergence of this field allows him to reconstruct the fate of hypothetical small circles drawn on the leaf. The construction of the
velocity at any point, however, admits nonlocal information; hence
this method is subject to error in much the same way as Green's if
the separation of sample points is not small with respect to any
variations in growth rate. It is possibly suggestive, in this

light, to note that the region where Erickson discovers anisotropy,
i.e. at the margin, is the very region where growth differentials
are high.

There are, however many biological systems where anisotropy is a
fundamental component of the growth. Indeed for any growth to be
regarded as a surface phenonmenon - and thus to fall into the
sphere or our current treatise - there must be a three dimensional
anisotropy favoring growth tangential to the surface over growth in
the normal direction. This phenomenon is exhibited in a study of
the development of the cerebral cortex by Smart (1973) in which the
neuron precursor population is shown to behave as a pseudostratified epithelium. Smart shows that all mitotic figures observed in
the developing tissue have planes of cleavage perpendicular to the
surface of the ventricle. Thus growth tangential to the ventricular surface is by cell division, growth perpendicular to the surface is by pseudostratification. The process of growth is therefore
directionally biased, and a three dimensional anisotropy is present. There is however no directional bias in the orientation of
mitotic figures between the different directions tangential to the
ventricular surface. Hence if we restrict ourselves to a 2-dimen-
sional surface viewpoint growth is isotropic.

In investigating the applicability of the isotropic assumption to a
particular system, it is worthwhile to analyse the biological mechanism responsible for the growth. Any clear directional bias in
this mechanism, for example growth by cell division oriented in one
specific direction, is evidence for anisotropy and argues against
the use of our isotropic growth model. On the other hand, in the
absence of any such evidence, isotropy is a natural assumption,
both as a mathematical simplification and, as we will now discuss,
as an expression of a unifying trend towards simplicity in biological development.

In describing biological growth it is essential to look at both the
process itself and also the system of control responsible for
directing the specific growth. It is a common observation that a
biological system knows what it wants to look like in advance and
grows accordingly. This pre-knowledge is an essential distinction
between biological and physical systems. It is also an expression
of the existence of a controlling supersystem encapsulating an

instruction set for a growth pattern which achieves the predesigned structure. This control process no less than the growth it engenders may be regarded as the product of a set of evolutionary pressures. One such pressure, discussed in Sauders and Ho (1981) is a principle of minimum increase in complexity in evolution. Applied to control processes we interpret this principle to say that where a number of different growth schemes are available to generate a given shape transformation, there is an evolutionary pressure towards the scheme with the least complex control mechanism.

Quantitative assessment of the complexity of a control regime without knowledge of the precise mechanism involved is difficult. For example a seemingly complex spatial pattern of growth may be greatly simplified when viewed from the perspective of concentrations of some controlling chemical obeying a particular reaction-diffusion equation. Another pattern which may be complex when seen as the result of a pattern of morphogen concentration may be simply controlled by some cell-automaton scheme. Without making assumptions about the control mechanism, therefore, any statements we make about the complexity of control necessary for a given growth regime must be regarded as suggestive rather that definitive.

A general growth pattern is a tensor field; it is necessary to specify at each point three quantities to specify this field - direction of maximum growth, its magnitude, and the ratio of maximum to minimum growths (the degree of anisotropy). To specify an isotropic growth pattern, however it is only necessary to set one quantity at each point - the magnitude of the growth. We have therefore achieved an economy in the control mechanism required to define the growth pattern. In some cases, however, this economy may be offset by an addition in complexity required to describe an essentially anisotropic process in terms of isotropic growth. An extreme example follows. To grow a rectangle with sides of length 1 and 2 from a square of side 1 one can use a uniform anisotropic growth, where the growth factor parallel to one side of the square is 2, and in the perpendicular direction is 1. While it is possible to achieve the same results with an isotropic growth regime, the pattern is far more complex.

In a similar way the growth with minimum Dirichlet integral is regarded as the least complex isotropic pattern, and therefore the

one whose control system would be the easiest to set up. Again
this assumption is made without knowledge of the actual mechanism
of control and admits to exception where some apparently complex
growth pattern is seen to be simple in terms of the mechanism
controlling the growth.

3.3 Some Properties of the Minimal Dirichlet Integral

In this section, we will discuss some of the mathematical properties of the minimum Dirichlet Integral. Specifically, we shall
show that in the case of axisymmetric surfaces S and T, the minimum
Dirichlet integral growth scheme is the axisymmetric growth scheme,
thus our principle is a genuine extension of the axisymmetric principle of section 2.2 above. We shall briefly discuss technical
conditions for two surfaces to be conformally equivalent.

Compatibility

Uniform growth: Where two surfaces are similar, the simplest
growth mapping would be expected to be uniform growth. Uniform
growth implies that λ is constant; hence $D[\lambda] = 0$ which, as
$D[\lambda] \geq 0$ by definition, is minimal. Hence the 'simplest', in our
technical sense, map between two similar surfaces, is indeed uniform growth.

Axisymmetric Growth: For our model to be compatible with the
axisymmetric model, it ought to reduce to it in the axisymmetric
case. We wish to prove, then, that for axisymmetric S and T $D[\lambda]$
is minimal when λ is axisymmetric.

Let ψ and χ be axisymmetric isotropic maps taking S and T respectively to the unit disc B in C. Then any $\varphi : S \to T$ may be
decomposed $\chi^{-1}\omega\psi$ where ω is a conformal map $B \to B$ (fig.
3.2.1). ω is therefore of the form

$$e^{i\Theta} \frac{z_0 - z}{\bar{z}_0 z - 1}$$

where $\Theta \in R$ and $z_0 \in \mathbb{C}$ such that $|z| < 1$

Let $\gamma(z)$ be the scale factor associated with the map $\psi^{-1}: B \to S$ and $\mu(z)$ the scale factor associated with $\chi^{-1}: B \to T$. The scale factor at z associated with ω is $|\omega'|$.

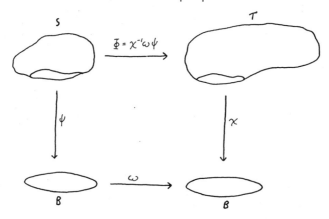

Figure 3.2.1 Conformal maps ψ and χ take surfaces S and T to the unit disc B. ω is a Moebis transform $B \to B$. Any conformal $\varphi = S \to T$ has the form $\chi^{-1}_{\omega\psi}$.

If $\omega_{z_0}(z) = \dfrac{z_0 - z}{\bar{z}_0 z - 1}$ we show first that

$$I_\omega = \iint_B \nabla \log(\upsilon(z)|\omega'(z)|\mu(\omega(z)))^2$$

is extremal at $\omega(z) = z$; i.e., $z_0 = 0$.

Let $z_0 = a + ib$ and $z = x + iy$ and
$$f(x, y, a, b) = \log(\upsilon(z)|\omega'(z)|\mu(\omega(z)))$$

then

$$I_\omega = \iint_B (\nabla f)^2$$

we evaluate

$$\frac{\partial I_\omega}{\partial a}\bigg|a = o, \; b = o$$

$$\frac{\partial I_\omega}{\partial a}\bigg|o, \, o. \; = \; 2\iint_B \nabla f\big|_{o, \, o} \cdot \nabla \frac{\partial f}{\partial a}\bigg|_{o, \, o}$$

now $f|o, \, o$ is axisymmetric; hence $\nabla f|o, \, o$ is antisymmetric in z.

Also $\frac{\partial f}{\partial a}|o, \, o$ is symmetric in z hence $\frac{\partial I_\omega}{\partial a}|o, \, o = 0$

similarly $\frac{\partial I_\omega}{\partial b}|o, \, o = 0$ so I_ω is stationary at $a = o, \; b = o$.

The symmetry of the system forces such a stationary point to be extremal. We require to show that this extremum is a minimum. We restrict ourselves to the simple situaiton illustrated in the text of a mapping between a symmetric surface and the unit disc; i.e., where $\mu = 1$.

Here

$$\frac{\partial^2 I_\omega}{\partial a^2} = \frac{\partial^2}{\partial a^2} \iint (\nabla \log(\nu|\omega'))^2$$

$$= 2\iint (\nabla \frac{\partial}{\partial a}\log(\nu|\omega'|))^2 + \nabla \log(\nu|\omega'|) \cdot \nabla \frac{\partial^2}{\partial a^2}\log(\nu|\omega'|)$$

now

$$\frac{\partial^2}{\partial a^2}\log(\nu|\omega^1|) = \frac{|\omega'|\dfrac{\partial^2|\omega'|}{\partial a^2} - (\dfrac{\partial|\omega'|}{\partial a})}{|\omega'|^2}$$

and

$$|\omega'| = \frac{1 - a^2 - b^2}{(ax + by - 1)^2 + (ay - bx)^2}$$

hence

$$\frac{\partial^2}{\partial a^2}\log\nu|\omega'|\bigg|_{a = 0, \; b = 0} = 2x^2 - 2y^2 - 2$$

and

$$\frac{\partial^2}{\partial a^2}\log(\nu|\omega'|) = \begin{pmatrix} 4x \\ -4y \end{pmatrix}$$

as log ν is radially symmetric:

$$\nabla\log\nu|\omega'|\Big|_{a = 0, b = 0} = F(x^2 + y^2) \begin{pmatrix} x \\ y \end{pmatrix} \text{ for some function } F$$

hence

$$\frac{\partial^2 I\omega}{\partial a^2} = 2\iint[(\nabla\frac{\partial}{\partial a}\log(\nu|\omega'|))^2 + F(x^2 + y^2)(4x^2 - 4y^2)]$$

$$= 2\iint(\nabla\frac{\partial}{\partial a}\log(\nu|\omega'|))^2 \geqslant 0$$

hence I_ω is minimal at $z = a + ib = 0$.

We have shown that the minimum Dirichlet Integral growth scheme
corresponds with more intuitive 'simplest growth schemes' in two
specific modelling problems: geometrically similar surfaces and
axisymmetric surfaces. The minimal Dirichlet integral growth will
be explicitly derived in an analytic example in section 3.3 below.
We now briefly mention the hitherto ignored conditions for two
surfaces to admit isotropic mappings one to another: that is for
two surfaces to be conformally equivalent.

The classification theorem for simply connected Riemann surfaces
(Farkas & Kra 1980) states that such a surface is conformally equivalent to exactly one of the unit disc, the unit sphere or the
plane. These mutually exclusive classes of surfaces are called
hyperbolic, elliptic and parabolic. In this thesis the surfaces we
shall deal with will be either elliptic (i.e., closed) or hyperbolic. In the sequel unless stated otherwise a surface is presumed
to be hyperbolic, and thus to admit a conformal mapping onto the
unit disc.

3.4 Minimum Dirichlet Integral as a Metric for Shape

Any parameter which attempts to quantify shape must be invariant to change in scale. Familiar two dimensional shape parameters include ratios such as perimeter^2/area, maximum diameter/minimum diameter; these ratios are scale invariant. For a parameter to quantify the intrinsic geometry, or shape, of a surface in three dimensions, there is a further requirement: it must in addition be invariant under isometric transformation of the surface. In this section we show that the minimum Dirichlet integral of scale factors is such a parameter and yields a natural measure of the intrinsic shape difference between surfaces.

Let $\underline{S}$ be the space of compact surfaces with piecewise continuous boundaries. We define the following equivalence relation on $\underline{S}$: if s_1 and s_2 ε $\underline{S}$ then s_1 $\sim$ s_2 if s_1 is geometrically similar to an isometry of s_2; i.e., if s_1 may be 'grown' from s_2 with uniform growth.

For two compact surfaces S and T, with piecewise continuous boundaries, we define

$$d(S, T) \text{ to be } : \sqrt{\min\iint_S (\nabla\log\lambda(\underline{s}))^2}$$

where $\lambda(\underline{s})$ is the scale factor at $\underline{s}$ of a conformal map S $\rightarrow$ T. We seek to show that d satisfies the triangle inequality. As $d(S, T) \geq 0$ by definition, d then defines a metric on the quotient space formed by making surfaces S_1 and S_2 equivalent if $d(S_1 \; S_2) = 0$.

Theorem 3.4.1 (triangle inequality for d).

If S_i, S_2, S_3 ε $\underline{S}$ the set of compact surfaces with piecewise boundaries then $d(S_1, S_2)$ $d(S_1, S_2) + d(S_3, S_2)$.

Proof

Let μ, ν and λ be the scale factors yielding minimum Dirichlet integral for maps $S_1 \rightarrow S_2$, $S_2 \rightarrow S_3$ and $S_1 \rightarrow S$ respectively. Let χ, ψ and φ be the conformal maps associated with these scale factors.

Firstly

$$d(S_2, S_1)^2 = \iint_S (\nabla \log \frac{1}{\mu(\chi^{-1}(\underline{s}))})^2$$

$$\equiv \iint_{S_2} (\nabla \log \frac{1}{\mu(\underline{s})})^2$$

by the invariance of the Dirichlet integral under conformal mapping
(Cohn 1967)

$$= \iint_{S_1} (\nabla \log \mu(s))^2 = d(S_1, S_2)^2$$

hence

$$d(S_2, S_1) = D(S_1, S_2)$$

now

$$d(S_1, S_3)^2 = \iint_{S_1} (\nabla \log \lambda(\underline{s}))^2$$

$$\leq \iint_{S_1} (\nabla \log \mu(\underline{s}) \nu(\chi(\underline{s})))^2 \text{ by definition of } \lambda$$

$$\equiv \iint_{S_1} (\nabla \log \mu(\underline{s})^2 + \iint_{S_1} (\nabla \log \nu(\chi(\underline{s})))^2 + 2\iint_{S_1} \nabla \log \mu \nabla \log \nu$$

$$\leq \iint_{S_1} (\nabla \log \mu(\underline{s}))^2 + \iint_{S_1} (\nabla \log \nu(\chi(\underline{s})))^2$$
$$+ 2\sqrt{\iint_{S_1} (\nabla \log \mu)^2 \iint_{S_1} (\nabla \log \nu)^2}$$

by Schwartz's Inequality

$$= \iint_{S_1} (\nabla \log \mu(\underline{s}))^2 + \iint_{S_2} (\nabla \log \nu(s))^2$$
$$+ 2\sqrt{\iint_{S_1} (\nabla \log \mu)^2 \iint_{S_2} (\nabla \log \nu)^2}$$

$$= (d(S_1, S_2) + d(S_2, S_3))^2$$

$$= (d(S_1, S_2) + d(S_3, S_2))^2 \qquad \text{Q.E.D.}$$

d is a metric on $\underline{T} = S/\sim$. It is thus reasonable to employ it as a
measure of distance on the space $\underline{T}$. The construction of $\underline{T}$ ensures
that surfaces which are isometric are in the same equivalence
class, and hence d = 0. Further, if t2 is merely a scaled up ver-
sion of t1 then t2 is in the same equivalence class as t1 and
d(t1, t2) = d(t1, t1) = 0. Hence d ignores difference in
scale and difference in geometry within isometry and measures only
intrinsic shape difference. Applied to a problem of biological surface growth, it is thus able to separate true differential growth
from 'uniform growth plus isometric defomration'.

Analytical Example

The truncated spheres of the tip growth model provide a convenient
analytic example to apply this metric. Let S be a sphere of radius
a truncated at z = k1a and T be a sphere of radius a truncated at
z = k2a. Then the simplest map φ is the axisymmetric map, which
has scale factor

$$\lambda = \frac{2aA}{2aA^2 + s(1 - A^2)}$$

where, using an anlogous argument to that of section 2.2 above.

$$A^2 = \frac{2(k_1 - k_1 k_2)}{(2 - k_1)k_2}$$

now if (σ, Θ) form an isothermic cordinate system on the sphere,

$$d(S, T) = \int\int \nabla(\log \lambda)^2 d\sigma d\Theta$$

$$\frac{d\sigma}{ds} = \frac{\sqrt{(\frac{dz}{ds})^2 + (\frac{dr}{ds})^2}}{r} = \frac{a}{2as - s^2}$$

so

$$d(S, T) = \int_0^{2\pi} \int_0^{k_1 a} [\frac{\partial}{\partial\sigma}\log\lambda]^2 d\sigma d\theta$$

$$= 2\pi \int_0^{k_1 a} [\frac{d}{ds} \log\frac{2aA}{2aA^2 + s(1 - A^2)}]^2 \frac{2as - s^2}{a} ds$$

$$= 2\pi[\frac{2(k_1 + k_2 - k_1 k_2)}{(k_2 - k_1)}\log\frac{2 - k_1}{2 - k_2} - (k_1 + k_2)]$$

Note (i)   This is symmetric in k_1 and k_2, hence $d(S, T) = d(T, S)$

(ii)   when $k_1 = k_2, d(S, T) = d(S, S) = 0$

(iii)   when $k_1 = 0$, $d(S, T) = 2 (2\log\frac{2}{2 - k_2} - k_2)$

This is the shape difference between a point and a truncated sphere. A flat disc may be grown uniformly from a point; so this is also the distance between a finite disc and a truncated sphere.

We note further that as k2 tends towards 2 the expression for d(S, T) tends to infinity. In the case where T is a complete sphere, i.e., when k2 = 2 our expression for d(S, T) becomes invalid. This is an expression of the fact that while a truncated sphere is conformally equivalent to a disc, an entire sphere is not.

3.5 Comparison with Other Dirichlet Problems

Many problems in mathematical physics may be formulated as variational problems: that is as the minimisation of some functional. This functional is often an energy term, and the variational principle regarded as a minimisation of free energy. The energy of a scalar potential field has the form of a Dirichlet integral: this type of integral is therefore frequently encountered in physics, and its properties widely studied. It is the purpose of this section to look at the relationship between the techniques of the Dirichlet problem in Physics and the surface growth analysis of this thesis. We first look at a typical physical Dirichlet problem, then a biological model applying the same analysis. Finally we look at the techniques of this chapter from the perspective afforded by these other models.

Our physical problem is that of deriving the equilibrium electrostatic potential distribution on a flat plate capacitor with a given potential applied to its boundary. A variational principle for this problem is to minimise the Dirichlet integral of the potential function subject to the boundary conditions. This is equivalent to minimising the potential energy of the field. The Euler Lagrange equation for this variational problem is the Laplace Equation $\nabla^2 \varphi = 0$; the solution of this partial differential equation with the prescribed boundary conditions yields the equilibrium potential distribution for the capacitor. Solutions to Laplace's equation are called 'harmonic functions'. The problem of minimising the Dirichlet integral over a region where the function value is specified on the boundary of the region is called the Dirichlet problem. Its solution is equivalent to finding a harmonic function taking the appropriate values on the boundary. This equivalence between variational problem and partial differential equation is called Dirichlet's Principle.

We have referred above to the fact that the Dirichlet integral is invariant under conformal mapping. Harmonic functions are therefore mapped into harmonic functions. For this reason, conformal mappings are a tool of great practical importance in two dimensional potential theory. If a mathematically awkward shape may be conformally mapped into a more easily treated shape, perhaps a disc or a half-plane, then the Dirichlet problem may be solved in the transformed plane, and the solution transformed back to give the solution to the original problem. Conformal mapping is here used as a mathematical trick for deriving a neat analytic solution to a problem, but is of no fundamental significance to the problem itself. The theoretical redundancy of conformal mapping in this role is evinced by the tendency for numerical methods of solving such problems to shun the conformal map and work on the Laplace's equation in the untransformed plane.

Classical potential theory is concerned with finding harmonic
functions with particular boundary values in a given region of
space. This is connected via Dirichlet's principle with minimising
the Dirichlet integral over the class of all fucntions with the
specified boundary conditions. Conformal mapping is a useful
technique, in two dimensions, of transforming problems into a
mathematically more succinct form. We now look at an application
of the above approach in biology.

A mapping which arises naturally in biology is the so-called
receptotopic map between peripheral receptor surfaces of the body
and corresponding regions of the central nervous system. In particular, the map arising from the connection of the retinal cells
of the visual system to the primary processing area of the CNS is
the subject of extensive research. Schwartz (1977) proposes a
geometric theory for such maps which models the system as a Dirichlet problem. His analysis of the mapping between retina and visual
tectum of the goldfish is based on the following assumptions. The
map is to be conformal, thus preserving local angles, a critical
functional requirement of a visual system; annular regions of the
retina are to map to rectangular regions of the tectum: this condition is based on observation and reflects the columnar nature of
the visual central nervous system. In addition Schwartz imposes a
'smoothest possible mapping' criterion by demanding that the integral of the magnification factor for the map be minimal. He treats
both the retina and the tectum as two dimensional surfaces.

The postulate of conformality implies that the retino-tectal map
may be expressed as a complex analytical function $f(z) = \varphi(x, y) +
i\psi(x, y)$. The magnification factor of the ampping is $|f'(z)|$.
Using the Cauchy Riemann equations (which may be invoked as f is
analytic)

$$\frac{\partial \varphi}{\partial x} = \frac{\partial \psi}{\partial y} \text{ and } \frac{\partial \varphi}{\partial y} = - \frac{\partial \psi}{\partial x}$$

$|f'(z)|$ may be written as $(\frac{\partial \varphi}{\partial x})^2 + (\frac{\partial \varphi}{\partial y})^2$ and hence

$$\iint |f'(z)| = \iint (\frac{\partial \varphi}{\partial x})^2 + (\frac{\partial \varphi}{\partial y})^2 = \iint (\nabla \varphi)^2$$

the Dirichlet integral of φ.

Minimisation of the Dirichlet integral of $\emptyset$ with respect to boundary conditions imposed by the shapes of corresponding regions of retina and visual tectum is equivalent via Dirichlet's Principle to solving Laplace's equation. The solution of Laplace's equation with the boundary conditions imposed by an annulus mapping to a rectangular region is the complex logarithm. Schwartz deduces the complex logarithm is an appropriate model for the retino-tectal map.

In this example, the variational formulation of the mathematical model came from consideration of the biology. Specifically, conformality (or local preservation of angles) derives from the functional requirements of the visual system. Minimal average magnification factor is adopted to express a 'smoothest possible map' hypothesis. The value of these rules in the view of Schwartz is that they comprise a set of minimal developmental rules in the following sense: they allow the structure of the receptotopic map to be determined by general mathematical principles rather than via biological encoding of detailed positional information. The quantity of information required to define the map is kept minimal and a parsimony, not only of the model but also of the developmental mechanism required to generate the system, is attained. We shall return to these themes shortly, but first we compare the Schwartz model with the 'simplest possible growth scheme' model of this thesis.

The models of this and the previous chapter require the simplest growth map to be conformal in order that growth rates may be expressed as a scalar field: that is locally growth is equal in all directions. It is therefore the isotropic property of the conformal map which is important to this model rather than its angle preserving property, which is emphasised in the Schwartz model. In both models a smoothest possible mapping function is required on grounds of developmental parsimony, and this generates a Dirichlet type problem.

Viewed from a biological angle, the models are similar, however mathematically there are some major differences. The Schwartz model is two dimensional, therefore his conformal mappings are the familiar conformal mappings of the complex plane, which are in fact the analytic functions. Our model maps Riemann surfaces in 3 dimensions; our conformal maps therefore are not necessarily complex analytical functions. Further, in our model $\mu = \log \lambda$ may not range freely over all sufficiently smooth functions but must generate the appropriate shape transformation. Instead of boundary conditions, we have restraints on admissible solutions. The classic Dirichlet approach is not applicable as this yields a minimum over all possible functions, and this minimal function may not generate the required shape change.

The models of this thesis and that of Schwartz diverge in their mathematical details. They do share, however, a common background philosophy: development along lines of minimal complexity. Saunders and Ho (1981) define a principle of 'minimal increase of complexity in evolution'. In line with this principle, an assumption of smoothest possible growth between two surfaces yields the least complex growth to account for observed shape change. We argue that such a growth scheme will arise preferentially from evolution, applying Saunders and Ho's principle. The smoothest growth assumption then plays a dual role: firstly as an instrument of parsimonious modelling, secondly as an expression of a general principle of minimal complexity in biological systems.

CHAPTER 4

CURVATURE OF THE FERRET BRAIN

In this chapter we measure the surface curvature of the ferret
brain. We analyse the changes in curvature during the process of
folding and interpret these changes in terms of different models of
folding.

We suggest two alternative views of cortical folding and derive expected curvature behavior of each. Our first model sees folding as
an isometric deformation imposed on uniform growth. The folding is
superimposed independent of the growth involved in cortical maturation. Geometrically, this may be seen as a two stage process: uniform growth followed by a pure non-growth 'bending' of the surface.
The effect of this type of folding on Gaussian curvature K is
clear. K has dimensions $(length)^{-2}$, thus uniform growth by a
scale factor L should cause K to decrease by a factor $1/L^2$. Gaussian curvature is a bending invariant, hence the 'bending' part of
the folding transformation has no effect on K. The expected curvature behavior with this model, then, is for Gaussian Curvature to
decrease as $1/L^2$.

A second model of folding has differential regional growth as an essential part of the folding process. The effect of this type of
folding on Gaussian curvature would be to cause local increase in K
at regions of relative growth.

In the discussion of their paper on cortical mapping, van Essen and
Maunsell (1980) identify Gaussian curvature as an important measure
of intrinsic differential growth. Based on the observation that it
is possible to draw flat maps of the folded cortex without too much
distortion, van Essen and Maunsell suggest that the folded cortex
is essentially isometric to the unfolded form. Their mapping process may be seen as 'In a sense, just a reversal of the developmental process'.

In this chapter, we shall measure the surface curvature of the ferret brain before and during the early stages of folding. Gaussian

curvature will be measured during the early stages of folding and any localised pattern of curvature increase detected. We will thus be able to pronounce on van Essen and Maunsell's speculations of limited increase in intrinsic curvature during folding.

4.1 Material & Methods

The ferret was chosen as the subject of this study because it has a small, simply folded brain, which is nonetheless representative of a broad class of carnivore brains. Neuron production in the ferret is prenatal, while folding is postnatal, a series covering the folding period may be obtained from a small number of litters. Further advantages of this animal are its comparative cheapness to obtain and maintain and its availability in laboratory strains.

Young postnatal ferrets were killed by an overdose of anesthetic and their brains perfusion fixed with Bouin's solution and, after removal, stored in 70% alcohol. They were then transported to the National Engineering Laboratory for Moire Fringe photography.

Two difficulties arise in the contouring of this type of object: firstly, since the surface of the brain tissue is translucent, a low contrast contour picture is formed; secondly, the pliant brain tissue is liable to distort during rotation. These problems are overcome by making an epoxy replica of the brain from a silicon rubber mould. This replica, after being lightly sprayed with matte white paint, provides high contrast and negligible distortions during rotation.

The centres of the dark and light bands on Figure 4.1.1 were taken as contour lines. Between 10 and 30 points from each contour were digitised using a magnetic digitising tablet. This provided x and y co-ordinates, z co-ordinates were determined from contour height.

The contour pattern was photographed and measurements made from an enlargement of the image. The example shown in Figure 4.1.1 is of a ferret brain at 8 days after birth. The use of a long focal length camera lens ensures equal magnification throughout the depth of the object. After the contour interval and magnification have been determined, surface co-ordinates are measured from the

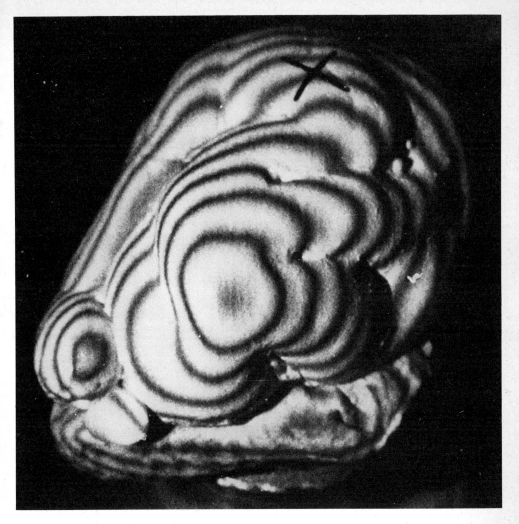

Figure 4.1.1 A Moire fringe photograph of an eight day ferret brain. Dark bands represent contours of equal height.

photograph. To obtain data over the entire surface, the object can be rotated and photographed in a number of positions. In the present example it was found that eight photographs (taken at angular intervals of 45 degrees) provided unobstructed views of every part of the surface together with sufficient information to relate one view to another.

Surface curvatures were estimated from the digitisations thus obtained by the indicatrix fitting method of appendix A. Surface curvature is displayed as the estimated indicatrix at data points. Gaussian and average curvatures are displayed by contour maps of least square best fit bicubic through estimated curvatures.

Splining is performed by NAG subroutines E02DAF and E02DBF, contour mapping by routines J06GFF and J06GZF.

4.2 Results and Interpretation

The cortex of a smooth brain is a convex surface. The curvature in all directions at a point on the surface has the same sign (positive if the surface is oriented such that its outward normal is external to the brain). The average surface curvature of a smooth brain is therefore positive throughout (figure 4.2.1a). In a folded brain, the tops of folds, or gyri, apparently retain similar curvature characteristics to the smooth brain: they are convex and have positive average curvature (figure 4.2.1b). At the base of sulci, however, the curvature in a direction perpendicular to the line of the sulcus is opposite in sign to the curvature of the cortex as a whole, and the curvature along the sulcus. Hence at sulci, average curvature is negative.

Average curvature, then, differentiates between the regions of the brain which can be regarded as gyral crests and those regions which can be regarded as sulcal troughs. We have gained nothing so far, as the observer can readily pick out these regions by inspection alone. We wish, however, to contrast average curvature, which is constrained to follow the sulcal pattern of the brain, with the Gaussian curvature which, a priori, is not so constrained. The average curvature of a surface reflects the configuration it has adopted in the embedding three dimensional space. It is closely connected, as we have seen, with the apparent shape or external appearance of the surface. Much variation in average curvature implies a somewhat folded surface, little variation in average curvature implies a smooth surface.

Gaussian curvature, on the other hand, reflects the intrinsic properties of a surface and is, to some extent, independent of the external appearance of the surface. Gaussian curvature is the product of maximum and minimum curvatures: a point with Gaussian curvature 1, for example, could have maximum and minimum curvatures k and $1/k$ for any $k \neq 0$; average curvature for this point could take any value from 1 up or from -1 down. The intrinsic properties of the surface, which are characterised by Gaussian curvature, are

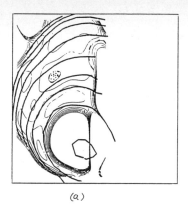

(a)

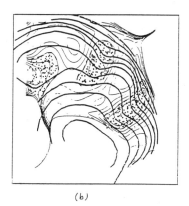

(b)

⟨⁚⁚⁚⟩ positive average curvature

Figure 4.2.1 Contour maps of average curvature are superimposed on brain surface contours taken from Moire photographs; (a) is a 1 day ferret brain, (b) is a six day ferret brain.

the same despite the vast difference in external appearance concomitant with these different average curvatures.

We do notice one option which is unavailable to the surface point with positive Gaussian curvature: it may never have principal curvatures of opposite signs. Similarly, whatever average curvature a point with negative Gaussian curvature may have, it may not have principal curvatures of the same sign. Regions of positive and negative Gaussian curvature distinguish two qualitatively different sets of points: those whose principal curvatures have the same sign (called elliptical points), and those whose principal curvatures have opposite signs (called hyperbolic points). (Points with zero Gaussian curvature are called parabolic points). These properties are intrinsic ones: under isometric transformation, elliptical points remain elliptical, hyperbolic points remain hyperbolic. The properties are also preserved by uniform growth plus isometric deformation and folding due to differential growth.

Figure 4.2.2a plots the estimated Dupin's indicatrix of points on the surface of a 1 day ferret brain. The Dupin's indicatrix is an ellipse for elliptical points, a pair of hyperbolae for hyperbolic points. The principal axes of the indicatrix are inversely proportional in length to the square root of the principal curvatures, and aligned in the direction of the principal curvatures. We note that the points on the surface of the unfolded brain are mainly elliptical. Some points near edges are apparently hyperbolic; however this is probably due to error in the numerical estimation routine which may be large when the points used for fitting curvatures are not evenly distributed.

Figure 4.2.2b plots the Dupin's indicatrix of a 6 day ferret brain. Points on gyri are in general still elliptical. Points inside folds, however, have now become hyperbolic, with a negative principal curvature aligned at right angles to the line of the fold and a positive curvature approximately aligned with the fold. This change in intrinsic type of the surface inside sulci during folding indicates that it is a non-isometric process,and therefore must involve differential growth. To say more about the pattern of differential growth, we look at the Gaussian curvature of the surface.

Figure 4.2.3 plots the Gaussian curvatures of similar views of the 1 and 6 day ferret brains respectively. We note first that there is a substantial increase in the magnitude of the Gaussian curvature during this period. This observation is at variance with what would be expected if folding consisted of uniform growth plus isometric deformation: in this case, Gaussian curvature should decrease as the inverse square of linear dimensions. Further, we note in the 6 day brain troughs of negative curvature as well as ridges of positive curvature, whereas in the smooth brain curvature is generally positive. This is all evidence for a differential growth theory of folding, as only differential growth can cause a change in sign of curvature.

Inspection of Figure 4.2.3 and further curvature maps of folded brains (figure 4.2.4) reveals that Gaussian curvature does indeed line up with the folding pattern of the brain. Gyri are in general areas of negative curvature. We now interpret this alignment of

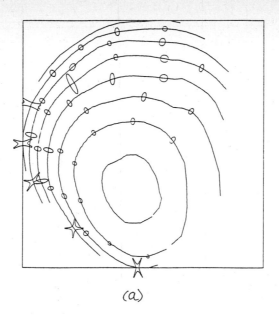

(a)

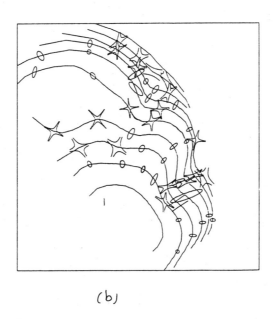

(b)

Figure 4.2.2 Dupin's indicatrix drawn at selected points on (a) a 1
day ferret brain (b) a 6 day ferret brain.

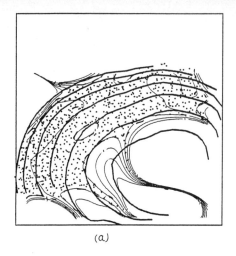

(a)

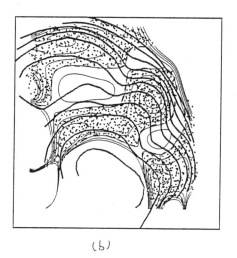

(b)

{image} positive Gaussian curvature

Figure 4.2.3 Gaussian curvature maps of (a) a 1 day ferret brain
(b) a 6 day ferret brain. The zero curvature contour
is boldly marked.

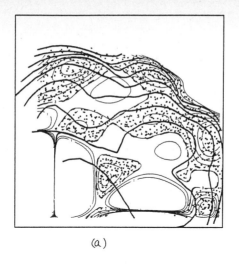

(a)

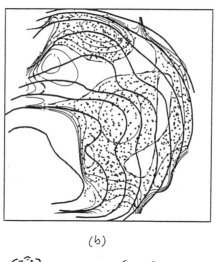

(b)

positive Gaussian curvature

Figure 4.2.4 Gaussian curvature maps of two further views of a six
day ferret brain.

curvature in terms of the differential growth experienced by the cortex during folding.

Gaussian curvature is a fundamental parameter in the study of the intrinsic differential geometry of a surface. Indeed if the Gaussian curvature of a surface is known, then its intrinsic geometry isdetermined. It is reasonable to hope that, knowing the Gaussian curvature of the brain, we should be able to make some useful inferences about its intrinsic geometry and about the intrinsic differential growth responsible for the geometry.

We observe (figure 4.2.3) that the Gaussian curvature of the unfolded 1 day old ferret brain is substantially less in magnitude than that of the folded 6 day brian. It is therefore a reasonable approximation to model the differential growth during folding as growth from a flat sheet to the eventual form. We introduce a further mathematical simplification by assuming that growth is isotropic. (See chapters 2 and 3 for further examples and discussion of this assumption.) We have remarked in chapter 2 that there are many isotropic (= conformal) maps between two surfaces; our maps of Gaussian curvature cannot therefore be expected to yield a unique differential growth field. We can, however, hope for some useful, if weaker, inforamtion about the growth field. We shall show that regions of positive Gaussian curvature correspond to regions where the growth rate function so defined has the super-mean-value property: that is the growth rate at a point exceeds the average growth rate around that point. This concept corresponds to the idea of a differential excess of growth.

Let $K(u, v)$ be the Gaussian curvature at point (u, v) on a surface $\underline{x}(u, v)$. Let a conformal map transform the x, y plane to the surface $\underline{x}(u, v)$ such that $\underline{x}(u(x, y), v(x, y))$ is the image of the point (x, y); let $\lambda(x, y)$ be the scale factor of this conformal map (i.e., $ds'^2 = \lambda^2 ds^2$). If E, F and G are the coefficients of the first fundamental form (2.3.2), $E = G = \lambda^2$, $F = 0$. When $F = 0$, the Gaussian curvature K of a surface can be expressed in terms of E and G as follows (Struik 1950)

$$K = \frac{1}{\sqrt{EG}} \left(\frac{\partial}{\partial x} \left(\frac{1}{\sqrt{E}} \frac{\partial \sqrt{G}}{\partial x} \right) + \frac{\partial}{\partial y} \left(\frac{1}{\sqrt{G}} \frac{\partial \sqrt{E}}{\partial y} \right) \right) \tag{4.2.1}$$

hence

$$K = -\frac{1}{\lambda^2}\nabla^2 \log\lambda \qquad\qquad (4.2.2)$$

Whence, while λ is finite, $\nabla^2 \log\lambda$ is opposite in sign to K. λ is the scale factor associated with some finite surface growth; we assume this growth was accomplished over time T by a field of relative elemental growth rates $\mu(x, y, t)$ (cf Erickson and Sax); if $h(x, y, t)$ is a line element then $dh/h = \mu dt$. Whence $\int\mu dt = \int\frac{dh}{h} = \log h - \log h_0 = \log\lambda$. $\log\lambda$ is equal to the total relative elemental growth rate at (x, y) integrated over time T; $\log\lambda$ is proportional to the average growth rate at (x, y). We have seen a similar use of the logarithm while averaging growth rates in section 2.2, $\log\lambda$ also plays an important role in the general growth model and shape metric of chapter 3.

Equation 4.2.2 may be applied to a model of an earlier section. In our model of the mouse cerebral vesicle (section 2.3), we derive the axisymmetric growth to form a truncated sphere of radius a from a unit flat disc (equation 2.3.4.):

$$\lambda(r) = 2aA/(1 + A^2 r^2)$$

Here A is a constant dependent on the plane of truncation.

$$1/\lambda = C + Dr^2, \text{ where } C = 1/2aA \text{ and } D = A/2a$$

Now

$$-\frac{1}{\lambda^2}\nabla^2 \log\lambda = \frac{1}{\lambda^2}\nabla^2 \log\frac{1}{\lambda} = (C+Dr^2)^2\,\frac{d^2 \log(C+Dr^2)}{dr^2} + \frac{1}{r}\frac{d}{dr}\log(C+Dr^2)$$

$$= (C + Dr^2)^2 (\frac{2DC - 2D^2 r^2}{(C + Dr^2)^2} + \frac{2D}{(C + Dr^2)})$$

$$= 4DC = \frac{1}{a^2}$$

which is the Gaussain curvature of a sphere of radius a.

Returning to look at equation 4.2.2 in a more general context, we
see immediately that any maximum of $\log\lambda$ must occur where $\nabla^2\log\lambda < 0$
and hence such a maximum may only occur in regions of positive
Gaussian curvature. Similarly, any minima of growth rate must occur at points with negative Gaussian curvature.

A function of one dependent variable $f(x)$ is convex if its second
derivative $\frac{d^2 f}{dx^2}$ is positive, concave if its second derivative is
negative. Analogous classes of functions of two dependent vari-
ables $g(x, y)$ are subharmonic functions, which have positive
Laplacian $\nabla^2 g$, and superharmonic functions, which have negative
Laplacian. A convex function $f(x)$ satisfies the one dimensional
sub-mean-value property:

$$f(x) \leq (f(x + h) + f(x - h))/2$$

a subharmonic function satisfies the corresponding bivariate sub-
mean value property (Beckenbach 1967)

$$g(x, y) \leq \frac{1}{2\pi}\int_0^{2\pi} g(x + r\cos\theta, y + r\sin\theta)d\theta$$

i.e., $g(x, y) \leq g_{ave}(x, y)$, the average value of g round a circle
centred (x, y). It can be further shown that

$$g(x, y) \leq \frac{1}{\pi r^2}\int_0^r\int_0^{2\pi} g(x + \rho\cos\theta, y + \rho\sin\theta)\rho d\rho d\theta$$

i.e., $g(x, y) \leq g_{AVE}(x, y)$, the average value of g over a cir-
cular disc centred (x, y).

Similarly, if g is superharmonic then $g \geq g_{ave}$ and $g \geq g_{AVE}$.

We have the following from equation 4.2.2: regions of positive
Gaussian curvature correspond to superharmonic growth rates, regions of negative Gaussian curvature correspond to subharmonic
growth rates. Hence in regions of positive curvature, growth rate

at a point is greater than the average growth rate near the point.
In regions of negative curvature, growth rate at a point is less
than the average growth rate near the point. In the sense thus
defined, areas of negative Gaussian curvature correspond to areas
of relatively low growth. We have noted above that gyri correspond
to regions of positive curvature on the ferret brain and that sulci
correspond to regions of negative curvature. Our analysis now lets
us identify gyri as regions of relatively high growth rate and
sulci as regions of relatively low growth rate. We infer that the
folding process involves a true outgrowth of the gyri, while surface growth is restricted at sulci.

There are many different isotropic maps between two surfaces. Our
analysis above, however, does not make any assumptions beyond isotropy, and hence applies to all such maps. Convexity is determined
by the sign of the second derivative; thus adding or subtracting a
straight line from a function does not alter its convexity
(straight lines have zero second derivative). In an analogous way,
using the Laplacian of a growth function to point out regions of
relative differential growth 'factors out' transformations of zero
Laplacian. These are exactly those transformations which map the
plane onto itself. We are therefore concentrating on the differential growth forced by the geometry of the surface, while ignoring
the larger scale differential growth on which these local variations are superimposed.

4.3 Discussion

In this study we analyse only the initial stage of folding: from 1
to 8 days post partem. During this period, the major patterns of
folding are set up: the sulci appear as shallow depressions, gyri
as gentle ridges. During the subsequent period, from 8 to about 20
days, the sulci deepen to form narrow crevasses, gyral crests
broaden to occupy most of the external surface of the brain. Here
we ignore the second stage of folding; we implicitly assume that
the process is a continuation of the patterns of differential
growth set up in the early stages.

For several reasons the first few days of folding constitute a particularly convenient subject for this study. The Gaussian curvature
analysis of this paper presupposes a model of the cerebral cortex
as a continuous twice differentiable mathematical surface. The surface we use as a model is the external surface of the cortex, measured by shadow Moire contouring. For our statements about differential growth of this surface to be relevant to the differential
growth of the cortex as a tissue, the physical structure of the cortex must be uniform in a transverse direction, or only slowly varying. Changes in cortical structure with depth are, however, toler-
ated. The key criterion is that differential growth observed at
the outermost surface of the brain may be interpreted as differential growth throughout the cortex, and not merely realignment of the
outer layer of cortex with respect to deeper layers. Companion histological studies (Smart 1984) show that before folding the cortical plate is a dense and uniform mass of cells. During the initial
stage of folding, while through the depth of the plate there is differentiation and maturation of neurons to form the different cortical layers, the transverse structure of the cortex remains largely
homogeneous. A transect of the cortex at the base of a sulcus remains similar to a transect taken at the crest of a gyrus. At this
stage of folding, then, the differential growth observed on the
outer surface of the brain accurately reflects the differential
growth undergone by the cortex throughout its depth. Concomitant
with folding, however, there is a differentiation in histological
structure beween the sulcal and gyral cortex. Cortex at the base
of sulci is eventually about a quarter of the thickness of cortex
at the crest of gyri. While the effects of this histological
change are not great up to 8 days, during the latter period of
folding histological variation through the cortex complicates the
relation between observed surface growth and tissue growth.

Further practical and mathematical considerations favour the analysis of the early days of folding. The shadow Moire contouring method used to acquire digitisations of the brain is only applicable
if an object may be illuminated from one angle and viewed from another. As the folds of the cerebral cortex close up, it becomes in-
creasingly difficult to illuminate and view the material within the
sulci. In practice it was found that an upper limit to the applicability of this digitisation technique was reached with the 10 day
ferret brain.

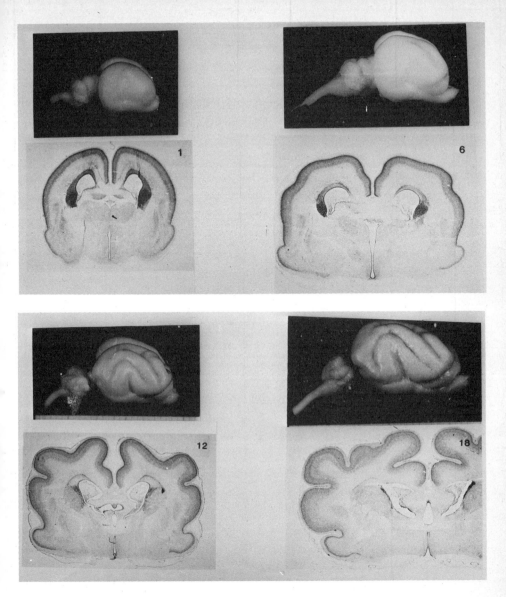

Figure 4.3.1 Pictures of the ferret brain and of coronal sections taken at 1,6, 12 and 18 days post conception.

The mathematical assumptions implicit in our surface model and the computational difficulties associated with numerical curvature estimation impose harsher restrictions on the applicability of the method. Our curvature estimation technique models the surface of the cortex as a smooth twice differentiable surface; the final form of a fold, however, is cusplike and plainly not differentiable. Before such analytical degeneracy of the surface is reached, however, computational difficulties preclude the application of our analysis. In practice there is an upper limit to the curvature which may be usefully estimated from a digitisation, and indeed the smaller the curvature to be estimated, the more accurate the numerical estimate. As the folds in the cortex close in, the curvature at the base of the sulcus grows large in the direction perpendicular to the sulcus. The ferret brain at older than 8 days begins to exhibit curvatures at the base of sulci sufficient to destabilise our numerical estimation techniques.

There is an underlying connection between the coincident degeneracy of the cortical surface as a mathematical entity and the disruption of the relationship between surface growth and cortical tissue growth. If we assume that the local average transverse tissue growth is a spatially smooth function over the cortex, then the onset of non-smooth features on the outer surface of the cortex must be associated with a relative realignment between outer and inner surfaces. The picture of folding we base our analysis on, then, is a spatially continuous twice differentiable cortical tissue growth. During the early stages of folding this growth is accurately portrayed by the growth of the cortical surface and assayed by a curvature function. During later stages of folding, the relationship between surface growth and cortical growth is disrupted by independent histological development at gyri and sulci; surface curvature is no longer a useful parameter of cortical growth.

By our study of the intact 3-dimensional geometry of the brain, we have shown a pattern of Gaussian curvature change during folding. This tells us first that folding is not merely uniform growth plus isometric deformation and that differential growth is in fact an essential part of the process. Further, the correlation between the Gaussian curvature increase and the folding pattern may be interpreted as preferential growth at gyri during the process of folding. Such a pattern of differential growth is interesting from the standpoint of theories on the functional significance of folding. We conclude by examining a possible relationship between functional subdivisions and differential growth in the cortex.

An external factor which might be expected to influence the folding of the cortex is pressure from the skull. By surgically removing portions of the developing cortex of sheep embryos, Barron (1950) relieves the pressure from the skull and finds the reduced cortex folds as normal. He concludes that 'the forces primarily responsible for folding in the cortex are primarily resident within the cortex.' Haddad et al. (1975) inject a neurotoxic agent (MAM) into ferrets during pre-natal development. The resulting neuron deficient brains exhibit abnormality in their folding, varying from complete lissencephaly, through regional lissencephaly to substantially normal brains. The extent of the disruption is related to the timing of the injection. This experiment, by reducing neuron numbers, interferes with the internal constitution of the cortex; the fact that the extent and pattern of folding is affected as a result suggests a strong link between the intrinsic growth of the cortex and its folding pattern.

A purely external explanation of the causes of folding would be expected to coincide, by and large, with the conservation of Gaussian curvature. Although some changes in the intrinsic structure of the surface could result from external mechanical pressure, the early stages of folding, when the cortex is apparently uniform, would naturallly appear to be isometric deformation (with no change in Gaussian curvature). The view of folding accompanied by systematic necessary differential growth which is the resault of our study of Gaussian curvature is therefore a picture of folding as a phenomenon intrinsic to the cortex.

The model put forward by Le Gros Clark (1942) postulates folding as a mechanical reaction to differences in physical structure of different functional areas of the cortex. The attraction of Le Gros Clark's model is that it presupposes, then utilises a link between the distribution of functional areas on the brain and its folding pattern. It is the difference in cytoarchitecture between regions with different functions which is assumed to generate the difference in physical structure which in the model drives folding. Certain folds do appear to adopt landmark positions with respect to functional areas. In primates, the central sulcus and the lunate sulcus reliably delimit the primary motor area and the primary visual area respectively (Connelly 1950). There is a substantial difference in thickness and therefore in physical properties between the visual area and the thicker surrounding cortex: a physical model such as Le Gros Clark's accounts for the accurate and reproducible alignment between cytoarchitecture and folding observed in this case. Welker & Campos (1963) ascribe a physiological significance to sulci in the somatic sensory region of different species in the family Procyonidae. Sulci are observed to maintain approximately constant position across the species with respect to the

sensory projection of the animal's body onto the cortex. For example, the Cornonal Sulcus of all the animals in this study lies between the projection of the head and the projection of the forelimbs. As we are now looking at subdivisions within the primary
sensory motor cortex, there is no histological difference between
regions; subdivisions are distinguished on physiological grounds
alone. A purely mechanical model of folding would not seem a satis-
factory medium for interpreting the alignment of folds with such apparently non-physical subdivisions.

Functional homology between sulci of different species is a pre-
condition for the interpretation of a number of studies by Radinsky
on brain evolution (Radinsky 1968, 1969, 1971, 1973). In Radinsky
(1968), for example, a relative enlargement, over an evolutionary
timescale, of the cornonal gyrus in fossil otters is interpreted in
terms of an elaboration of the somatic sensory projection of the
otter's head. Such an interpretation is crucially dependent on a
stable functional homology between sulci; particularly so as the
fossil data is not susceptible to physiological corroboration.

A theoretical objection to the proposed constancy of the coronal
sulcus as a boundary between the head and forelimb sensory representation on the cortex is that there need be no difference in cytoarchitectonic structure between these regions; thus, to a model
with a mechanical bias, there is no reason for their boundaries to
align with sulci. Such an argument treats the cortex solely in
terms of its physical properties: elasticity, density, volume. In
an attempt to introduce some of the more detailed structure of the
cortex into the model one might speculate as follows. Perhaps
neurons receiving sensory projections from the head require strong
intracortical connections with neighbouring neurons also receiving
input from the head, while they require rather weaker intracortical
communication with neighbouring neurons which receive projections
from the forelimbs. Similarly, neurons receiving forelimb projections might require a multiplicity of connections to allow integration with other forelimb projections, while requiring fewer connections with neurons receiving projectiont from the head. The development of such a pattern of intercellular communcation would be expected to exhibit local excess growth of tissue at strongly connected regions and locally deficient growth between such strongly
connected regions, due respectively to local excess of neuropil and
local dearth of neuropil. Thus sulci, which we have observed to

develop along lines of locally deficient growth, would tend to correspond to boundaries between strongly connected regions of cortex.

4.4   The nearest plane region to a given surface

In this section we identify the plane region which is nearest in shape (using the metric of chapter 3) to a given surface.

<u>Definition</u>   Let S be a surface which admits a conformal map φ : $R \to S$ for some bounded plane region R such that the scale factor λ of φ is continuous non-zero and finite on ∂R, the boundary of R. We define the <u>associated plane map</u> to φ to be the map ω with scale factor ν such that $\log\nu$ is harmonic on R and $\log\nu = \log\lambda$ on ∂R.

<u>Lemma 4.4.1</u> ωR is flat.
<u>proof</u>   As $\log\nu$ is harmonic, by 4.2.2   R has zero Gaussian Curvature and hence can be viewed as a plane region.

<u>Lemma 4.4.2</u>   Let μ be the scale factor of the map $\psi = \varphi\omega^{-1}$: $(\omega R) \to S$, $\log\mu = 0$ on $\partial(\omega R)$
<u>proof</u>   for $r \in R, \mu(\omega r) = \frac{\lambda(r)}{\mu(r)}$ hence $\log\mu = \log\lambda - \log\nu$ but for $r \in \partial R$ $\log\lambda = \log\nu$, hence $\log\mu = 0$.

<u>Lemma 4.43</u>   For two plane regions R_1 and R_2, let φ_1 : $R_1 \to S$ and φ_2 : $R_2 \to S$ be conformal maps with scale factors λ_1 and λ_2 and associated plane maps ω_1 and ω_2. $\omega_1 R_1 = \omega_2 R_2$ and $\varphi_1\omega_1^{-1} = \varphi_2\omega_2^{-1}$ (to within isometry).
<u>proof</u>   Let $\psi_1 = \varphi_1\omega_1^{-1}$ and $\psi_2 = \varphi_2\omega_2^{-1}$, then $\chi \equiv \psi_2^{-1}\psi_1$ is a conformal map between $\omega_1 R_1$ and $\omega_2 R_2$. Let μ be the scale factor of χ. As $\omega_1 R_1$ and $\omega_2 R_2$ are both flat by lemma 4.4.1, $\log\mu$ is harmonic (from 4.2.2) but on $\partial(\omega_1 R_1)$, $\log\mu = 0$ hence $\log\mu = 0$ on $\omega_1 R_1$. Hence χ has unity scale factor and is an isometry; thus $\psi_1 = \psi_2$ to within isometry.

<u>Definition</u>   If S is a surface which admits a conformal map from a plane region φ : $R \to S$ with scale factor λ such that λ is continuous non-zero and finite on ∂R and if ω is the associated plane map to φ, we call (ωR) the associated plane region to S.

Theorem 4.4.4 Let S be a surface with associated plane region T, let R be another plane region conformally equivalent to S, then $d(S, T) \leq d(S, R)$ - here $d(., .)$ is the minimum Dirichlet integral metric of chapter 3. Further, the map yielding the minimal Dirchlet integral is the map whose scale factor is constant on the boundary.

proof Let φ be a conformal map $R \rightarrow S$ with scale factor λ, let ω be the associated plane map : $R \rightarrow T$, let ν be the scale factor of ω. Let μ be the scale factor of the map $\psi = \varphi\omega^{-1}$: $T \rightarrow S$. For $r \in R$, $\lambda(r) = \mu(\omega r)\nu(r)$ whence $\log\lambda = \log\mu + \log\nu$ so

$$\iint_R (\nabla\log\lambda)^2 = \iint_R (\nabla\log\mu)^2 + \iint_R (\nabla\log\nu)^2 + 2\iint_R \nabla\log\mu \cdot \underline{\nabla}\log\nu$$

$$= \iint_T (\nabla\log\mu)^2 + \iint_R (\nabla\log\nu)^2 - 2\iint_R \log\mu\nabla^2\log\nu$$

$$+ 2\int_{\partial R}\log\mu\underline{\nabla}\log\nu \cdot \underline{n}ds$$

Now $\nabla^2\log\nu = 0$ on R and $\log\mu = 0$ on ∂R so we have:

$$\iint_R (\nabla\log\lambda)^2 = \iint_T (\nabla\log\mu)^2 + \iint_R (\nabla\log\nu)^2$$

hence

$$\iint (\nabla\log\lambda)^2 \leq \iint (\nabla\log\mu)^2$$

this is true for all $\varphi : R \rightarrow S$ hence

$$d(S, T) \leq d(S, R)$$

If $R = T$ we have shown that the map yielding the minimum Dirchlet integral is ψ : the map with constant scale factor at the boundaries.

Corollory 4.4.5 If S is a surface with associated plane region T and R is any plane region conformally equivalent to S then

$$d(S,R)^2 = d(S, T)^2 + d(R, T)^2$$

proof From the proof of 4.4.4 if φ is any map $R \rightarrow S$ and if all other symbols retain their meaning.

$$\iint (\nabla \log \lambda)^2 = \iint (\nabla \log \mu)^2 + \iint (\nabla \log \nu)^2$$

hence

$$\min_{\emptyset : R \to S} \iint (\nabla \log \lambda)^2 = \iint (\nabla \log \mu)^2 + \min_{\emptyset : R \to T} \iint (\nabla \log \nu)^2$$

$$\Rightarrow d(S, R)^2 = d(S, T)^2 + d(R, T)^2$$

Example

In chapter 3 we derived an axisymmetric map between 2 axisymmetric surfaces. In particular if one surface is a disc, we have an axisymmetric map from the disc to our second surface. Symmetry prescribes constant boundary conditions for this map; it is thus the minimal Dirichlet integral map. The closest plane surface to an axisymmetric surface is thus a disc.

Practical application of this result might include the drawing of optimal flat maps of curved objects, e.g., physiological maps of brains. Many manufacturing processes involve stretching flat panels to make curved surfaces: here we have identified, in one sense, the optimal flat panel to start with.

4.5 Conclusions

The geometry of a growing surface imposes certain restraints on the form of the growth. Any conformal growth on the plane, for example, must have a growth rate μ which satisfies Laplace's equation $\nabla^2 \mu = 0$; solutions of this equation are exactly the analytic functions. If the conformal growth maps one particular simple connected bounded region into another, then the geometry of these regions constrains the growth. Any simply connected region may be conformally mapped onto the unit disc (Riemann's Mapping Theorem). Given φ and ψ which map our regions onto the unit disc, any conformal map between the regions has the form $\psi^{-1}\omega\varphi$ where ω is a Moebius transform. The geometry of the regions dictate growth to within a Moebius Transform.

In chapter 4, we looked at conformal mappings from a planar region
to a general surface. In this case, the equation relating surface
geometry to growth is (4.2.2)

$$\nabla^2\mu = Ke^{2\mu} \qquad\qquad \mu = \log\lambda,$$

where K is the Gaussian Curvature of the surface. If Φ is a conformal mapping between these surfaces, then its growth rate μ satisfies the above equation.

If φ maps the plane region to a unit disc, then any conformal map
between plane region and surface may be written $\Phi\varphi^{-1}\omega\varphi$ where ω is a
Moebius transform. Whence φ is unique to within Moebius transform:
any properties of Φ which are not affected by Moebius transform, we
may hope to derive from surface geometry. One such property is the
super-mean-value property: the function value at a point is
greater than the mean function value in a circle round the point.
Regions with the super-mean-value property correspond to regions of
negative Laplacian of growth rate. If f represents a growth rate,
then compounding f with a Moebius transform is equivalent to adding
a function g with zero Laplacian. Hence the super-mean-value property is invariant under Moebius transformation. It is for this
reason that the super-mean-valued property of growth rate is an at-
tribute which is determinable from Gaussian Curvature.

In section 3.4 we defined a metric for the difference in intrinsic
shape between two surfaces. As a measure of shape, this metric had
to be invariant under magnification, as a measure of intrinsic surface shape it had to be invariant under isometry. The metric used
was $d(S,T) = \min \iint (\nabla\mu)^2$ where is growth rate for conformal mappings between the surfaces S and T.

Throughout the essay, a modelling theme has counterpointed the metric motif. We have repeatedly looked at isotropic models of surface growth; this because isotropy is sufficient for any growth between topologically equivalent finite surfaces, and is a natural
simplifying modelling assumption. In the case studies of sections
2.2 and 2.3, axisymmetry was a second condition: this defined a
unique growth model. In chapter 3, a replacement principle was
that the growth map should have minimal Dirichlet integral of

growth rate. The natural growth model thus defined is the smoothest isotropic growth permitted by the geometry of the two surfaces.
The metric for intrinsic geometry mentioned above may thus be expressed as 'the smoothness of the smoothest isotropic growth between two surfaces.'

A similar relationship between parameter and model appears in the
interpretation of Gaussian curvature in chapter 4. An isotropic
model of growth and a flat approximation of the unfolded cortex
allow us to apply the mathematics of section 4.2 and claim the
super-meanvalue property for growth rate at presumptive gyri, and
the sub-meanvalue property for growth rates at sulci.

At first glance, it might appear that we should be able to derive a
growth map by solving equation (4.2.2), numerically or otherwise.
In the case of mapping from a disc to a surface with constant curvature (e.g., a sphere) this is certainly true. For surfaces with
non-constant curvature, however, knowing $K(x, y)$ in (4.2.2) necessi-
tates a knowledge of $u(x, y)$ and $v(x, y)$: the growth map is hence
already known. To reverse the process and write an equation for
the growth factor requires the surface to be presented in terms of
an isometric coordinate net. Once such a coordinate system is
known, however, a conformal map to the plane is simply one which
maps the surface coordinate net to an isometric net on the plane
(e.g., the Cartesian grid). The scale factor for this map may be
obtained directly and an equation relating curvature to growth is
redundant.

The key problem in determining conformal growth between two surfaces is thus the derivation of an isometric coordinate net on the
surfaces. One isometric net is that formed by the principal curvature lines on the surface. An objective of further numerical studies would be to derive an isometric parametrisation by principal
curvatures of a digitised surface. Such a curvature-implicit parametrisation could be obtained by fitting (with appropriate smooth-
ing) to digital curvature estimates obtained using the methods of
Appendix A. An appropriate first step in the study of this problem
would be to analyse a homologous problem in curve fitting: the definition of a curve from a curvature/arclength profile estimated
from a digitisation. This is an interesting problem in its own
right.

REFERENCES

Adams, J. A. (1975), "The intrinsic method for curve definition", Computer Aided Design 7:243.

Ariens Kappers, C. U. Huber, G. and E. C. Crosby (1936), The Comparative Anatomy of the Nervous System of Vertebrates, Including Man (New York: Macmillan).

Beckenbach, E. F. (1967), "Inequalities in the differential geometry of surfaces", in Inequalities, ed. O. Shisha (New York: Academic Press).

Bookstein, F. L. (1978), The Measurement of Biological Shape and Shape Change (Berlin: Springer-Verlag).

Bookstein, F. L., R. E. Strauss, J. M. Humphries, B. Chernoff, R. L. Elder, and G. R. Smith (1982), 'A comment on the uses of Fourier methods in systematics', Syst. Zool 31:85.

Campos, G. B. and W. I. Welker (1976), "Comparisons between brains of a large and a small hystriomorph rodent - capybara hydrochoerus and guinea-pig cavia - neocortical projection regions and measurements of brain subdivisions", Brain Behaviour and Evolution, 13:243.

Chi, J. G. (1977), "Gyral development", Annals of Neurology, 1:86.

Clark, W. E. Le Gros (1945), "Deformation patterns in the cerebral cortex" in Essays on Growth and Form, ed. W. E. Le Gros Clark (Oxford: Clarendon Press).

Connolly, C. J. (1950), External Morphology of the Primate Brain (Springfield: Thomas).

Crowther, R. A., D. J. Rosier, and A. Klug (1970), "The reconstruction of a 3 dimensional structure from its projections and its applications to electron microscopy", Proc. Roy. Soc. Lond. A, 317:319

Dimitrov, D. S., G. A. Georgiev, N. G. Stoicheva, T. T. Traykov (1982), "Dynamics of viscoelastic spherical Membranes - the balloon model of the alveolus", J. Theor. Biol., 96:517.

Erickson,R. O. (1966), "Relative elemental rates and anisotropy of growth in area", J. Exp. Bot., 17:390.

Erickson, R. O. and K. Sax (1956), Proc. Am. Phil. Soc. 100:487.

Evrard, P., V. S. Caviness, J. Prato-Vinas, and G. Lyon (1978), "The mechanism of arrest of neuronal migration in the Zellweger malformation: a hypothesis based on cytoarchitectonic analysis", Acta. Neuropath. Berl. 41:109.

Falk, D. (1978), "Brain evolution of old world monkeys" Am. J. P. Anth. 48(3): 315.

Farkas, H. M. and I. Kra (1980), "Riemann Surfaces", New York: Springer-Verlag.

Fuchs, H., Z. M. Kedem, and S. P. Uselton (1977), "Optimal surface reconstruction from planar contours", Comm. Assoc. Comp. Mach. 20:693.

Goodwin, B. C. (1977), "Mechanics fields and statistical mechanics in developmental biology", Proc. Roy. Soc. Lond. 199:407.

Green, P. B. (1965), "Pathways of cellular morphogenesis", J. Cell. Biol. 27:343.

Green, P. B. (1969), "Cell morphogenesis", Ann Rev. Plant. Physiol. 20:365.

Green, P. B. (1976), "Growth and cell pattern formation on an axis", Botan. Gazette, 137:187.

108

Greenspan, H. P. (1976), "On the growth and stability of cell cultures and solid tumors", J. Theor. Biol. 56:229.

Haddad, R. K., A. Y. Rabe, R. Dumas (175), "CNS birth defects", Comparative Pathology Bulletin 7:2.

Hejnowicz, Z. (1982), "Vector and scalar fields in modelling of spatial variations of growth rates within plant organs", J. Theor. Biol. 96:161.

Hejnowicz, Z. and J. Nakielski (1979), Acta. Soc. Bot. Pol. 48:423.

Helms, L. L. (1969), Introduction to Potential Theory (New York: Wiley-Interscience).

Humphries, J. M. X., et al. (1981), "Multivariate discrimination by shape in relation to size", Syst. Zool. 30:291.

Jerison, H. J. (1963), "Interpreting the evolution of the brain", Hum. Biol. 35:203.

Jones, D. S. and B. D. Sleeman 91983), Differential Equations and Mathematical Biology (London: Allen and Unwin).

Korr, H. (1980), Proliferation of Different Cell Types in the Brain (Berlin: Springer-Verlag).

Levin, D., N. Papamichael, and A. Sideris (1976), "The Bergman kernal method for the numerical conformal mapping of simply connected Domains", J. Inst. Maths. Applics. 22:171.

Levitt, P. and P. Rakic (198), "Immunoperoxidase localization of glial fibrillary acidic protein in radial glial cells and actrocytes of the developing rhesus monkey brain", J. Comp. Neurol. 193:815.

Love, A. H. and R. L. Somorjai (1982), "Differential geometry of proteins: a structural and dynamical representation of patterns", J. Theor. Biol. 98:189.

Meadows, D. M., W. O. Johnson and J. B. Allen (1970), "Generation of surface contours by moire patterns", Applied Optics 9:942.

Pal, T. K. and A. W. Nutbourne (1977), "Two dimensional curve synthesis using linear curvature elements", Computer Aided Design 9:77.

Preston, F. W. (1953), "The shape of birds' eggs", Auk, 70:160.

Radinsky, L. B. (1968), "A new approach to mammalian cranial analysis, illustrated by examples of prosimian primates", J. Morph. 124:167.

Radinsky, L. (1971), "An example of parallelism in carnivore brain evolution", Evolution, 25:518.

Radinsky, L. (1973), "Evolution of the canid brain", Brain Behaviour and Evolution, 7:169.

Radinsky, L. (1974), "The fossil evidence of anthropoid brain evolution", An. J. Phys. Anthrop. 41:15.

Rakic, P. (1981), "Neuronal glial interaction during brain development", Trends in Neurosciences 4:184.

Richards, O. W. and A. J. Kavanagh (1943), "The analysis of the relative growth gradients and changing form of growing organisms: illustrated by the tobacco leaf:, Amer. Nat. 77:385.

Richards, O. W. and A. J. Kavanagh (1945), "The analysis of growing form" in Clark and Medawar (eds.) Essays on Growth and Form, Oxford: Clarendon Press, pp. 188.

Richman, D. P., R. M. Stewart, J. W. Hutchinson, V. S. Caviness (1975), "Mechanical model of brain convolutional development", Science, Vol. 189:18.

Ritter, R. and R. Schettler Koehler (1983), "Curvature measurement by Moire effect", Experimental Mechanics 23:165.

Da Rivva, Ricci D. and B. Kendrick (1972), "Computer modelling of hyphal tip growth in fungi", Can. J. Bot. 50:2455.

Sacher, G. A. (1970), "Allometric and factorial analysis of brain structure in insectivores and primates" in Noback and Montagna (eds.) Advances in Primatology (New York: Appleton Century Crofts), pp. 245-287.

Salmon, G. (1912), "A treatise on the analytic geometry of three dimensions", (London: Longmans Green & Co.).

Saunders, P. T. and M. W. Ho (1981), "On the increase in complexity in evolution, the relativity of complexity and the principle of minimum increase", J. Theor. Biol. 90(4):515.

Schechter, A. (1978), "Linear blending of curvature profiles", Computer Aided Design 10:100.

Scheiben, K. J. (1979), "Coherent optimal correlation - new method of cranial comparison", Am. J. P. Anth. 51(2):235.

Schwartz, E. L. (1977), "The development of specific visual connections in the monkey and the goldfish: outline of a geometric theory of receptotopic structure", J. Theor. Biol. 69:655.

Schwartz, E. L. (1980), "Computational anatomy and functional architecture of striate cortex - a spatial mapping approach to perceptual coding", Vision Research 20(8):645.

Silk, W. K. and R. O. Erickson (1978), "Kinematics of hypocotyl curvature", Am. J. Botany, 65:310.

Silk, W. K. and R. O. Erickson (1979), "Kinematics of plant growth", J. Theor. Biol. 76:481.

Sinai, G., D. Zaslavsky, and P. Golamy (1981), "The effect of soil surface curvature on moisture and yield - Beer Sheda observation", Soil Science 132:367.

Skalak, R., G. Dasgupta, and M. Moss (1982), "Analytic description of growth", J. Theor. Biol. 94:555.

Smart, I. H. M. (1969), "The method of transformed co-ordinates applied to the deformations produced by the walls of a tubular viscus on a contained body: the avian egg as a model system", J. Anatomy 104:507.

Smart, I. H. M. (1973), "Proliferative characteristics of ependymal layer during early development of mouse neocortex", J. Anatomy 116:67.

Smart, I. H. M. (1983), "Three dimensional growth of the mouse isocortex", J. Anatomy 137:683.

Smart, I. H. M. (1986), "Gyrus formation in the telencephalic cortex of the ferret", (in preparation).

Smart, I. H. M. and G. M. McSherry (1982), "Growth patterns in the lateral wall of the mouse telencephalon II", J. Anatomy 134:415.

Strauss, R. E. and F. L. Bookstein (1982), "The truss: body form reconstruction in morphometrics", Syst. Zool. 31:113.

Struik, D. J. (195), "Lectures on classical differential geometry" (Cambridge: Addison-Wesley).

Thompson, D'Arcy (1942), "On growth and form", Cambridge University Press.

Todd, P. H. (1983), "A geometric model for the cortical folding pattern of simple folded brains", J. Theor. Biol. 97:529.

Todd, P. H. (1984), "The shape of birds' eggs", J. Theor. Biol. 106:239.

Todd, P. H. and I. H. M Smart (1982), "Growth patterns in the lateral wall of the mouse telencephalon: III Studies of the chronologically ordered column hypothesis of isocortical histogenesis" J. Anatomy 134:633.

Van Essen, D. C. and J. M Maunsell (1980), "2-dimensional maps of
    the cerebral cortex", J. Comp. Neurol. 191(2):255.

Walker, G. F. and C. J. Kowalski (1971), "A two dimensional
    coordinate model for the quantification, description,
    analysis, prediction and simulation of craniofacial growth",
    Growth 35:191.

Welker, W. I. and G. B. Campos (1963), "Physiological significance
    of sulci in somatic sensory cerebral cortex in mammals of the
    family Procyonidae", J. Comp. Neurol. 120:19.

Xenofos, S. S. and S. H. Jones (1979), "Theoretical and practical
    applications of Moire topography", Phys. Med. Biol. 24:250.

Younker, J. L. and R. Ehrlich (1977), "Fourier biometrics:
    harmonic amplitudes as multivariate shape descriptors", Syst.
    Zool. 26:336.

Appendix A   Numerical Surface Curvature

Two different potential methods are analysed. In one method, a
quadric surface is fit to 9 data points. The curvature of the
quadric at the centre point is then taken as an estimate of the
curvature of the digitised surface at that point. The second
method also works from 9 data points, but fits the Dupin's indicatrix of the surface to linear curvatures in 4 directions
through the centre point. The Dupin's indicatrix yields a full
description of surface curvature at the centre point.

In this section we first define the two numerical methods. In
order to compare the performance of the methods, we require a metric for surface curvature. A suitable metric is defined; we can
then apply both methods to known surfaces and use our metric to derive an error.

Quadric Surface Method

Let 9 distinct points x_{ij} $1 \leq i \leq 3$, $1 \leq j \leq 3$ lie on a surface
P. We estimate the curvature of P at x_{22} by the curvature at x
of the unique quadric surface Q which passes through all x_{ij}. In
special cases this quadric may degenerate to a pair of parallel
planes. This eventuality may be precluded by ensuring that data
points from three parallel planes are present. The general equation of a quadric surface is

$$ax^2 + by^2 + cz^2 + 2eyz + 2fxz + 2gxy + 2px + 2qy$$
$$+ 2rz + d = 0 \tag{A1}$$

We transform coordinates so that the point x_{22} is the origin by
constructing x_k as follows:

Let $x_k = x_{1k} - x_{22}$ for $1 \leq k \leq 3$,
let $x_4 = x_{21} - x_{22}$ and $x_5 = x_{23} - x_{22}$
and let $x_k = x_3(k-5) - x_{22}$ for $6 \leq k \leq 8$.

Our quadric now passes by construction through the origin, so $d = 0$.

We now assume $a \neq 0$ and divide (4.4.1) by a and substitute the x_k to obtain the following set of linear equations:

$$\underline{A} \cdot \underline{X} = \underline{B} \text{ where} \tag{A2}$$

and

$$\underline{A} = \begin{bmatrix} y_1^2 & z_1^2 & y_1z_1 & x_1z_1 & x_1y_1 & x_1 & y_1 & z_1 \\ y_2^2 & z_2^2 & y_2z_2 & x_2z_2 & x_2y_2 & x_2 & y_2 & z_2 \\ \cdot & \cdot & \cdot & \cdot & \cdot & \cdot & \cdot & \cdot \\ \cdot & \cdot & \cdot & \cdot & \cdot & \cdot & \cdot & \cdot \\ y_8^2 & z_8^2 & y_8z_8 & x_8z_8 & x_8y_8 & x_8 & y_8 & z_8 \end{bmatrix}$$

and

$$\underline{X} = \begin{bmatrix} b/a \\ c/a \\ e/a \\ f/a \\ g/a \\ p/a \\ q/a \\ r/a \end{bmatrix} \qquad \underline{B} = \begin{bmatrix} x_1^2 \\ x_2^2 \\ \cdot \\ \cdot \\ \cdot \\ \cdot \\ x_8^2 \end{bmatrix}$$

Equation (A2) may be solved for $\underline{X}$ by some standard numerical technique (e.g., Gaussian elimination) to yield coefficients a, b, c, e, f, g, p, q, r.

Having found the quadric Q which passes through the 9 points, we
need to determine the curvature of Q at the origin. It is
convenient to work in homogeneous coordinates (x, y, z, w). The
equation of the quadric is then:

$$(x \quad y \quad z \quad w) \begin{bmatrix} a & g & f & p \\ g & b & e & q \\ f & e & c & r \\ p & q & r & 0 \end{bmatrix} \begin{bmatrix} x \\ y \\ z \\ w \end{bmatrix} = 0$$

or $x^T Q x = 0$ (A3)

To determine the curvature of Q we make use of the following result
(Willmore 1950). If coordinate axes are chosen with origin at a
point on a surface, with z axis aligned with the surface normal at
that point, and with x and y axes along the directions of principal
curvature at the point, then as z tends to 0 the surface tends to
the paraboloid

$$k_1 x^2 + k_2 y^2 = 2z$$

where k_1 and k_2 are the principal curvatures at the point.

We first rotate the axes so the surface normal at the origin is
parallel to the z axis. The normal at the origin is parallel to
(p, q, r) in the old coordinate system; so we generate a new system

$$(x' \quad y' \quad z' \quad w') = (x \quad y \quad z \quad w) \underline{D}$$

so that z' is parallel to (p q r).

$$\underline{D} = \begin{array}{c|c} C & 0 \\ \hline 0 & 1 \end{array}$$

where C is the matrix of direction cosines of the appropriate x, y, z transformation.

Under this coordinate transformation, quadratic form Q transforms to

$$Q' = D^T Q D \qquad (A4)$$

Let $Q' = \begin{bmatrix} a' & g' & f' & 0 \\ g' & b' & e' & 0 \\ f' & e' & c' & r' \\ 0 & 0 & r' & 0 \end{bmatrix}$

As z tends to O, the surface $x'^T Q' x' = O$ tends to the paraboloid

$$Ax^2 + By^2 + 2Cxy = 2z$$

where

$$A = -a'/r', \quad B = -b'/r', \quad C = -g'/r'.$$

Principal curvatures and directions of principal curvature now correspond to the eigenvalues and eigenvectors of the 2 by 2 matrix

$$\begin{bmatrix} A & C \\ C & B \end{bmatrix}$$

These eigenvalues and eigenvectors may be obtained by rotating the x'y' plane by an angle θ where $\tan\theta = 2C/(A - B)$.

Dupin's Indicatrix Method

At a point on a surface whose principal curvatures are k_1 and k_2, the Dupin's Indicatrix is defined to be the locus of points (x, y) such that

$$k_1 x^2 + k_2 y^2 = \pm 1 \qquad\qquad (A5)$$

This locus is either

(i)   an ellipse if $k_1 k_2 > 0$

(ii)   a pair of hyperbolae if $k_1 k_2 < 0$.

Euler's theorem on curvature (Struik p. 81) states that the normal curvature in direction α is

$$k = k_1 \cos^2 + k_2 \sin^2 \alpha$$

Now the line in direction $y = \tan\alpha$ intersects the conic (A5) in the points

$$x = \frac{\pm \cos\alpha}{\sqrt{k_1 \cos^2\alpha + k_2 \sin^2\alpha}} \qquad y = \frac{\pm \sin\alpha}{\sqrt{k_1 \cos^2\alpha + k_2 \sin^2\alpha}} \qquad (A6)$$

Thus the radius of the conic in the direction α is

$$\frac{1}{\sqrt{k_1 \cos^2\alpha + k_2 \sin^2\alpha}} = \frac{1}{\sqrt{k}} \qquad\qquad (A7)$$

Hence the radius of the Dupin's indicatrix in any direction is the square root of the radius of normal curvature of the surface in the corresponding direction.

Our numerical procedure will involve:

(i)   estimating the direction of the surface normal and estimat-
        ing normal curvatures in a number of directions.

(ii)   fitting a Dupin's Indicatrix to vectors of magnitude $1/\sqrt{k}$ in
        the directions of the curvatures.

(iii)   finding the principal axes of the indicatrix.

When the indicatrix is expressed in terms of its principal axes,
its coefficients are used as estimates for the principal curvatures
of the surface. The directions of its principal axes are taken as
estimates for the directions of principal curvature.

We now look at the process in more detail.

Given 3 points $\underline{x}$-1, $\underline{x}$0, $\underline{x}$1 we define tangent and curvature
vectors associated with the circle passing through the points. $\underline{T}$
is the unit vector tangential to the circle at $\underline{x}$0 (or a unit vector along the line if the points are collinear). $\underline{K}$ is a vector
parallel to the interior normal to the circle at $\underline{x}$0 with magnitude the inverse of the radius of the circle (or the 0 vector if
the points are collinear).

If $\underline{u} = \underline{x}$-1 $-$ $\underline{x}$0 and $\underline{v} = \underline{x}$-1 $-$ $\underline{x}$0, then the centre of the
circle through $\underline{x}$-1, $\underline{x}$0, $\underline{x}$1 is (a, b) where

$$a = \frac{\underline{u}^2 v_1 - \underline{v}^2 u_1}{2|\underline{u} \wedge \underline{v}|} \qquad\qquad b = \frac{\underline{v}^2 u_2 - \underline{u}^2 v_2}{2|\underline{u} \wedge \underline{v}|} \qquad\qquad (A8)$$

Hence

$$\underline{K} = \frac{1}{a^2 + b^2}\binom{a}{b} \qquad \text{and } \underline{T} = \frac{(\underline{u} \wedge \underline{v}) \wedge \underline{k}}{|(\underline{u} \wedge \underline{v}) \wedge \underline{k}|} \qquad\qquad (A9)$$

Given 9 points x_{ij} $1 < i < 3$, $1 < j < 3$ from a digitisation of a
surface P, we select 4 sets of points

```
S0 = x21, x22, x23
S1 = x31, x22, x13
S2 = x11, x22, x33
S3 = x12, x22, x32
```

For each triplet of points S_i, we define tangent and curvature vectors $\underline{T}_i$ and $\underline{K}_i$ as above.

Each pair of vectors $\underline{T}_i$, $\underline{T}_j$ $i \neq j$ defines a plane tangent to the pair of circles S_i and S_j and a unit vector perpendicular to this plane

$$\underline{N}_{ij} = \frac{\underline{T}_i \wedge \underline{T}_j}{|\underline{T}_i \wedge \underline{T}_j|} \tag{A10}$$

We estimate the surface normal by the average of these normals

$$\underline{n} = \frac{\Sigma \underline{N}_{ij}}{|\Sigma \underline{N}_{ij}|} \tag{A11}$$

To estimate the normal curvature of surface P in the directions of the circles S_i we make use of Meusner's Theorem (Struik 1980 p. 76)). This theorem relates the curvature K of an arbitrary section of a surface to the curvature k of a normal section in the same direction by the equation

$$K = K\cos\Theta$$

where Θ is the angle between teh normals of the two curves. Hence an estimate for the normal curvature in direction $\underline{T}_i$ is

$$K_i = \underline{K}_i \cdot \underline{n} \tag{A12}$$

To fit the Dupin's indicatrix, we first transform coordinates so that the plane perpendicular to $\underline{n}$ is the x, y plane.

Let $\underline{X}_1 = (X_i, Y_i) = \frac{1}{\sqrt{|K_i|}}\underline{T}_i$

If k_i was the true surface curvature in direction $\underline{T}_i$, and the Dupin's indicatrix were the locus of points:

$$Ax^2 + By^2 + 2Cxy = \pm\, 1$$

then the following should hold:

$$AX_i^2 + BY_i^2 + 2CX_iY_i = \text{sgn}(k_i) \text{ for } 0 \leq i \leq 3$$

We wish to find a 'best fit' indicatrix, hower to 4 points which do not necessarily lie on the same locus. One possible definition of 'best fit' is to minimise the function:

$$\sum_i [AX_i^2 + BY_i^2 + 2CX_iY_i - \text{sgn}(k_i)]^2 \tag{A13}$$

The minimum of (A13) may be shown to be the solution of the matrix equation

$$
\begin{bmatrix}
\sum_i X_i^4 & \sum_i X_i^2 Y_i^2 & \sum_i X_i^3 Y_i \\
\sum_i X_i^2 Y_i^2 & \sum_i Y_i^4 & \sum_i X_i Y_i^3 \\
\sum_i X_i^3 Y_I & \sum_i X_i Y_i^3 & \sum_i X_i^2 Y_i^2
\end{bmatrix}
\begin{bmatrix}
A \\ B \\ 2C
\end{bmatrix}
=
\begin{bmatrix}
\sum_i X_i\,\text{sgn}(k_i) \\
\sum_i Y_i\,\text{sgn}(k_i) \\
\sum_i X_i Y_i\,\text{sgn}(k_i)
\end{bmatrix}
$$

Solving this matrix equation yields values A, B, C for the coefficients of the indicatrix.

Principal axes, and principal values of the coefficients are now eigenvectors and eigenvalues of the matrix

$$
\begin{bmatrix}
A & C \\
C & B
\end{bmatrix}
$$

These eigenvalues may be found by performing the appropriate rotation of the x, y plane as described for the quadric fitting method.

A Metric for Surface Curvature

Average and Gaussian curvature are scalars. The relative performance of our two numerical curvature methods for measuring these
scalar curvatures may be assayed by comparing estimated versus actual curvature for known surfaces. Taken as a whole however, surface curvature is a quadratic form. It is necessary therefore to
define a suitable metric before a comparison may be made.

Let L and M be two real symmetric 2 by 2 matrices representing the
Dupin's indicatrices of two surface curvatures. We define a metric
d such that

$$d(L, M) = \rho(L - M)$$

where $\rho(L - M)$ is the spectral radius of $L - M$. This is the spectral norm on the space of real symmetric 2 by 2 matrices. If
$L - M = \begin{bmatrix} \alpha & \gamma \\ \gamma & \beta \end{bmatrix}$ then $\rho(L - M) =$

$$\frac{1}{2} \left[|\alpha + \beta| + \sqrt{(\alpha - \beta)^2 + (2\gamma)^2} \right] \tag{A14}$$

We now look at some of the properties of d and interpret how pertinent they are to quantifying surface curvature.

Let $L = \begin{bmatrix} A & O \\ O & B \end{bmatrix}$

expressed in coordinates parallel with the principal axes of the indicatrix.

Let $M = \begin{bmatrix} C & O \\ O & D \end{bmatrix}$

expressed in a coordinate system lined up with its own principal
axes, not necessarily the same axes as those of form L. Let α be
the angle between the coordinate systems.

In the coordinate system of form M, form L is

$$
\begin{bmatrix} \cos\alpha & \sin\alpha \\ -\sin\alpha & \cos\alpha \end{bmatrix} \begin{bmatrix} A & O \\ O & B \end{bmatrix} \begin{bmatrix} \cos\alpha & -\sin\alpha \\ \sin\alpha & \cos\alpha \end{bmatrix} \tag{A15}
$$

$$
= \begin{bmatrix} A\cos^2\alpha + B\sin^2\alpha & (B - A)\cos\alpha\sin\alpha \\ (B - A)\cos\alpha\sin\alpha & A\sin^2\alpha + B\cos^2\alpha \end{bmatrix} \tag{A16}
$$

whence

$$
d(L,M) = [|(A +B) - (C + D)| + (A - B)^2 + (C - D)^2 \\ -2(A - B)(C - D)\cos2\alpha] \tag{A17}
$$

Some properties of $d(L, M)$ follows:

(i)   If the indicatrix corresponding to M is a circle, then $C = D$ and $d(L, M) = \max\ [|A - C|,\ |B - C|]$, which is independent of α.

(ii)   If $\alpha = O$ then $d(L, M) = \max\ [|A - C|,\ |B - D|]$

(iii)   If $\alpha = \frac{\pi}{2}$ then $d(L, M) = \max\ [|A - D|,\ |B - C|]$

We now assume coordinates whose origin lies on our surface such that the z axis is parallel to the surface normal at the origin and the x and y axes lie along the principal axes of curvature.

By Euler's theorem the curvature of the normal section through the surface in a direction specified by a unit fector $\underline{x} = (x, y)$ is

$$
k = k_1 x^2 + k_2 y^2
$$

$$
= x^T L x
$$

where L is the matrix representing the indicatrix of the surface at the origin.

The difference in curvatures in direction $\underline{x}$ between surfaces with indicatrices L and M is

$$x^T L x - x^T M x = x^T (L - M) x$$

L and M and hence L - M are symmetric, so $L - M = A^T A$ for some A.

Now $\rho(L - M) = \rho(A^T A) = ||A^2||$ where $||.||$ is the Euclidean Norm. $||A|| = \max \underline{x}^T A^T A \underline{x}$ for $|\underline{x}| = 1$

hence

$$\rho(L - M) = \max \underline{x}^T (L - M) \underline{x} \text{ for } |\underline{x}| = 1$$
$$= \text{maximum difference in curvature between normal sec-}$$
tions of the two surfaces.

In (A13) we fit the Dupin's indicatrix to a number of curvature vectors by minimising the function

$$F = \sum_i (A X_i^2 + B Y_i^2 + C X_i Y_i - \text{sgn}(k_i))^2$$

$$= \sum_i (X_i^T L X_i - \text{sgn}(k_i))^2$$

Now if $X_i = x_i / \sqrt{|k_i|}$ and if l_i is the curvature of L in direction x_i then

$$F = \sum (\frac{l_i}{|k_i|} - \text{sgn}(k_i))^2$$

$$= \sum (\frac{l_i - k_i}{|k_i|})^2$$

which is the relative difference between the curvature of L in direction x_i and the measured curvature in that direction.

Having defined a suitable metric for surface curvature, we may now compare the two numerical methods outlined above.

Comparison and Analysis of Numerical Methods

In order to compare the performance of the two numerical surface
curvature techniques described above, we apply them to sets of
points taken from known surfaces and compare the estimated
curvature with the true surface curvature. To compare curvatures,
we use the metric of equation (A17). It is also useful to compare
the accuracy of estimates of scalar quantities Gaussian Curvature
and Average Curvature.

Figure A1 graphs the results of computer simulations designed to
compare the accuracy of the two methods.

Data points $\underline{x}_{ij}$ $1 \leq i \leq 3$, $1 \leq j \leq 3$ are taken from a paraboloid.
Simulated data error is introduced by perturbing the data set in
the following way:

$$\underline{x}_{ij}' = \begin{bmatrix} x_{ij} + \varepsilon p_{ij} \\ y_{ij} + \varepsilon q_{ij} \\ z_{ij} \end{bmatrix}$$

where p_{ij} and q_{ij} are drawn from uniform random distributions
on $[-1, 1]$ and $\varepsilon > 0$ is a prescribed constant. The curvature
estimated numerically for the points x_{ij}' may then be compared
with the true curvature fo the paraboloid (determined analytically)
at x_{22}.

This simulation is repeated a large number of times and for a range
of values of ε. Graphs of the average curvature error encountered
during the simulation yield a good indication of the behavior of
the numerical methods under varying quantities of data error.
Figure A1 graphs the errors in different types of curvature
produced by each method. Overall difference in surface curvature,
as measured by the spectral radius metric of (A17), is graphed in
figure A1a. Gaussian Curvature error is depicted in figure A1b,
average curvature error in figure A1c.

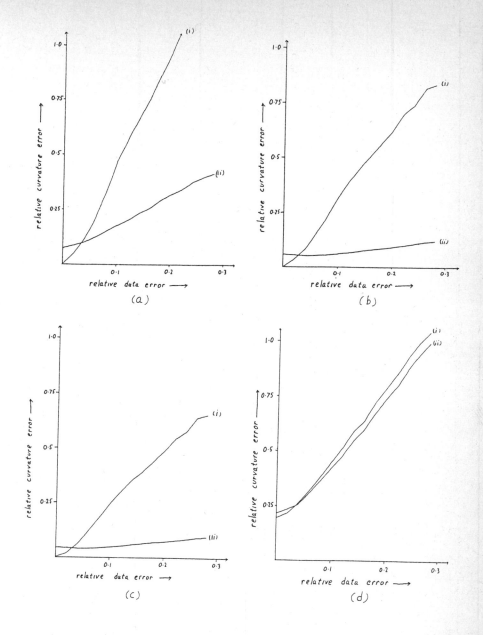

Figure A1.   Graphs of relative error in curvature estimate against
relative data error introduced to known surfaces in a
computer simulation.   (a) error in surface curvature
measured by the spectral radius metric; (b) error in
Gaussian curvature; (c) error in Average Curvature.   In
each case (i) is curvature estimated by quadric fitting, (ii) is curvature estimated by the Dupin's indicatrix method; (d) a comparison between curvature estimated by (i) the least square best fit Dupin's indicatrix, and (ii) by the indicatrix derived from the alternative fitting algorithm.

The quadric surface fitting technique is exact for a paraboloid surface. Thus with zero or low data error, is very accurate. However
as data error increases, the technique rapidly becomes unstable in
the simulation and experiences explosive error growth. The Dupin's
Indicatrix method is exact only for spheres; it is therefore not as
accurate as the quadric technique when applied to exact data from a
quadric surface. Curvature error, however, appears to increase lin-
early with data error and to remain manageable. It would thus
appear to be the more practicable of the two techniques to apply to
real data.

In order to picture the significance of typical numerical curvature
errors, in figure A2a the Dupin's indicatrix of a number of points
on a paraboloid are plotted; in A2b the Dupin's indicatrix of
numerical curvature estimates from exact data are plotted for
comparison; in figure A2c an error has been incorporated in the
data from which the numerical estimate has been derived. Figure
A3a plots the Dupin's indicatrix at a number of points from a
hyperbolic paraboloid. A3b plots numerical estimates from exact
data, A3c plots numerical estimates from data with error for this
surface.

When looking at the Dupin's indicatrix, it must be remembered that
the major axes of the indicatrix are inversely proportional in
length to the square root of the principal curvatures in those
directions. The direction of minimum curvature is thus along the
long axis of the indicatrix. In general the larger the indicatrix,
the less the curvature and the flatter the surface. Although a
large hyperbola and a large ellipse are very different in geometry,
the curvatures which these indicatrices describe are both
relatively flat, and are rather similar.

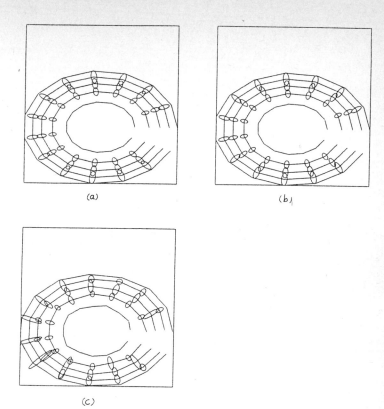

Figure A2.   (a) The Dupin's indicatrix of a number of points on a
paraboloid, superimposed on controus of the surface;
(b) the indicatrices estimated from exact data taken
from the paraboloid; (c) the indicatrices estimated
from data points with error superimposed.

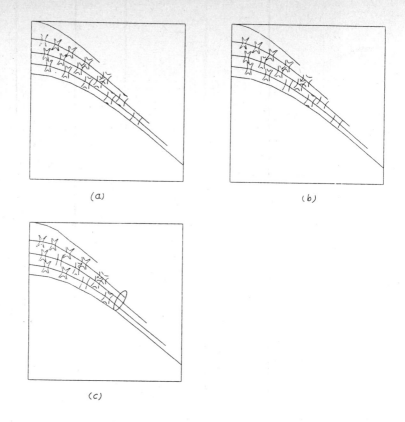

(a)

(b)

(c)

Figure A3.   (a) The Dupin's indicatrix of a number of points from a
hyperbolic paraboloid superimposed on a contour map of
a portion of the surface; (b) Dupin's indicatrices estimated from exact data; (c) Indicatrices estimated from
data with superimposed error.

Linking mathematics and biology

Journal of

Mathematical Biology

Subscription Information:
ISSN 0303-6812   Title No. 285
1986, Vol. 24 (6 issues)
For Subscribers outside North America: DM 596,- plus carriage charges.
For Subscribers in USA, Canada and Mexico:
US $ 237.00 (includes postage and handling).

For sample copies or instructions for authors, please contact one of the addresses listed below

The **Journal of Mathematical Biology** serves as a meeting ground for mathematics and biology. It publishes papers ranging from those which provide new theoretical formulations of current biological issue, to those which use substantive mathematical techniques in solving biological problems. It is must reading for the biologist interested in theoretical questions, and for the mathematician seeking new problems and new inspiration from biological applications.
Among the fields addressed regularly in the journal are population genetics, ecology, epidemiology, demography, physiology, cell biology, morphogenesis, chemistry, and physics.

Selected articles from recent issues:

W. L. Keith, R. H. Rand: 1:1 and 2:1 phase entrainment in a system of two coupled limit cycle oscillators.
S. Karlin, S. Lessard: On the optimal sex-ratio: A stability analysis based on a characterization for one-locus multiallele viability models.
S. Ellner: Asymptotic behavior of some stochastic difference equation population models.
O. Dlakmann, H. J. A. M. Heijmans, H. R. Thieme: On the stability of the cell size distribution.
A. Hunding: Bifurcations of nonlinear reaction-diffusion systems in oblate spheroids.
J. K. Hale, A. S. Somolinos: Competition for fluctuating nutrient.
M. Bertsch, M. E. Gurtin, D. Hilhorst, L. A. Peletier: On interacting populations that disperse to avoid crowding: The effect of a sedentary colony.
Y. Iwasa, E. Taramoto: Branching-diffusion model for the formation of distributional patterns in populations.

Springer-Verlag
Berlin Heidelberg
New York Tokyo

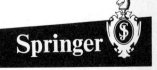

Springer

Bio-mathematics

Managing Editor: **S.A.Levin**

Editorial Board: **M.Arbib, H.J.Bremermann, J.Cowan, W.M.Hirsch, J.Karlin, J.Keller, K.Krickeberg, R.C.Lewontin, R.M.May, J.D.Murray, A.Perelson, T.Poggio, L.A.Segel**

Springer-Verlag
Berlin Heidelberg
New York Tokyo

Volume 17

Mathematical Ecology

An Introduction

Editors: **Th.G.Hallam, S.A.Levin**

1986. Approx. 87 figures. Approx. 495 pages
ISBN 3-540-13631-2

Contents: Introduction. – Physiological and Behavioral Ecology. – Population Ecology. – Communities and Ecosystems. – Applied Mathematical Ecology. – Subject Index.

Volume 16

Complexity, Language, and Life: Mathematical Approaches

Editors: **J.L.Casti, A.Karlqvist**

1986. XIII, 281 pages. ISBN 3-540-16180-5

Contents: Allowing, forbidding, but nor requiring: a mathematic for human world. – A theory of stars in complex systems. – Pictures as complex systems. – A survey of replicator equations. – Darwinian evolution in ecosystems: a survey of some ideas and difficulties together with some possible solutions. – On system complexity: identification, measurement, and management. – On information and complexity. – Organs and tools; a common theory of morphogenesis. – The language of life. – Universal principles of measurement and language functions in evolving systems.

Volume 15

D.L.DeAngelis, W.Post, C.C.Travis

Positive Feedback in Natural Systems

1986. 90 figures. Approx. 305 pages. ISBN 3-540-15942-8

Contents: Introduction. – The Mathematics of Positive Feedback. – Physical Systems. – Evolutionary Processes. – Organisms Physiology and Behavior. – Resource Utilization by Organisms. – Social Behavior. – Mutualistic and Competitive Systems. – Age-Structured Populations. – Spatially Heterogeneous Systems: Islands and Patchy Regions. – Spatially Heterogeneous Ecosystems; Pattern Formation. – Disease and Pest Outbreaks. – The Ecosystem and Succession. – References. – Appendices A to H.

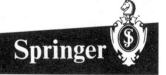

Springer